D1233827

A Primer of Biomechanics

Springer
New York
Berlin
Heidelberg
Barcelona
Budapest
Hong Kong
London
Milan
Paris
Singapore
Tokyo

George L. Lucas, M.D.
Francis W. Cooke, Ph.D.
Elizabeth A. Friis, Ph.D.

QP
303
L82
1999
Davis

A Primer
of Biomechanics

Illustrations by Danielle Y. Chinn

With 146 Illustrations

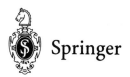 Springer

George L. Lucas, M.D.
Professor and Chairman, Department of
  Surgery, Division of Orthopaedic
  Surgery, University of Kansas School
  of Medicine, Wichita, KS 67214, USA

Francis W. Cooke, Ph.D.
Research Director, Orthopaedic
  Research Institute, Inc., Via Christi
  Regional Medical Center–St. Francis
  Campus
Research Professor, Department of
  Surgery, Division of Orthopaedic
  Surgery, University of Kansas School
  of Medicine, Wichita, KS 67214, USA

Elizabeth A. Friis, Ph.D.
Research Scientist, Orthopaedic Research
  Institute, Inc., Via Christi Regional
  Medical Center–St. Francis Campus
Research Instructor, Department of
  Surgery, Division of Orthopaedic
  Surgery, University of Kansas School
  of Medicine, Wichita, KS 67214,
  USA

Danielle Y. Chinn
Graphic Designer/Illustrator, dc design

Library of Congress Cataloging-in-Publication Data
Lucas, George L.
    A primer of biomechanics / George L. Lucas, Francis W. Cooke,
  Elizabeth A. Friis.
        p.   cm.
    Includes bibliographical references and index.
    ISBN 0-387-98456-9 (softcover : alk. paper)
    1. Human mechanics.   2. Orthopedics.   I. Cooke, Francis W.
  II. Friis, Elizabeth.   III. Title.
  QP303.L83   1998
  612.7′6—dc21   97-48865

Printed on acid-free paper.

© 1999 Springer-Verlag New York, Inc.
All rights reserved. This work may not be translated or copied in whole or in part with-out the written permission of the publisher (Springer-Verlag New York, Inc., 175 Fifth Avenue, New York, NY 10010, USA), except for brief excerpts in connection with re-views or scholarly analysis. Use in connection with any form of information storage and retrieval, electronic adaptation, computer software, or by similar or dissimilar methodol-ogy now known or hereafter developed is forbidden.
The use of general descriptive names, trade names, trademarks, etc., in this publication, even if the former are not especially identified, is not to be taken as a sign that such names, as understood by the Trade Marks and Merchandise Marks Act, may accordingly be used freely by anyone.
While the advice and information in this book are believed to be true and accurate at the date of going to press, neither the authors nor the editors nor the publisher can accept any legal responsibility for any errors or omissions that may be made. The publisher makes no warranty, express or implied, with respect to the material contained herein.

Production coordinated by Impressions Book and Journal Services, Inc., and managed by Terry Kornak; manufacturing supervised by Thomas King.
Typeset by Impressions Book and Journal Services, Inc., Madison, WI.
Printed and bound by Maple-Vail Book Manufacturing Group, York, PA.
Printed in the United States of America.

9 8 7 6 5 4 3 2 1

ISBN 0-387-98456-9   Springer-Verlag   New York Berlin Heidelberg   SPIN 10659576

This book is dedicated to the residents in orthopaedic surgery—past, present, and future—who have studied our syllabus on biomechanics, worked through the demonstration problems, and worked with us in the laboratory.

Preface

A substantial knowledge of biomechanics and biomaterials is essential for today's orthopaedic surgeon. Unfortunately, most of us do not come from an engineering background, and much of the writing about biomechanics is difficult for us to understand. This is particularly true when a mathematical formula is utilized because, even if one has taken calculus in college, such skills are quickly forgotten if not used regularly. A few simple formulas are essential for clarity, and remembering a few basic ones can come in handy when taking the Orthopaedic In-Training Examination or perhaps Part I of the American Board of Orthopaedic Surgery Examination, but none of the formulas in this book require anything beyond a rudimentary recollection of basic algebra.

In an effort to understand how and why a patient's bone broke, how to repair such a fracture, or why a certain repair technique did not succeed, orthopaedic surgeons constantly employ a knowledge of and appreciation for mechanics, forces, force dimensions, velocity, and numerous other concepts related to biomechanics. Thus we need to understand as clearly as possible, without resorting to complex analyses or mathematical calculations, as much about biomechanics as is practical. This book provides fundamental knowledge about the subject in a highly readable and understandable fashion. We have attempted to demystify the subject of biomechanics while providing the student, orthopaedic resident, or even practicing orthopaedist with basic concepts that will heighten their understanding of clinical situations. One of our basic techniques of teaching orthopaedics is to encourage residents to relate what they have read in texts or journals to specific patients they have seen. Reaching back into one's mind to recall how a similar patient was treated is much more effective than trying to remember something read out of context in a textbook on fractures, for example. By providing brief, clinical vignettes to introduce various subtopics of biomechanics, reader interest and focus is, in our view, significantly enhanced. We hope that readers will find this approach a refreshing way to come to grips with what is sometimes considered a "dry" subject.

GEORGE L. LUCAS, M.D.
FRANCIS W. COOKE, PH.D.
ELIZABETH A. FRIIS, PH.D.

Acknowledgments

This book, like all others, has been both a labor of love and a test of our will. Also, like all other books, this work is not exclusively the product of the authors, and we acknowledge the assistance and support of many others. We are especially grateful to the following persons:

Our families for their patient understanding and forbearance during this period

Dustan Hahn, former research assistant in the Orthopaedic Research Institute, with whom the idea was first discussed

Juanita Ridgeway and Rita Baker, our secretaries, for help with secretarial details

The hospital volunteers who helped with proofreading, typing, and photocopying

Via Christi Regional Medical Center (St. Francis) for facility and personnel support

Charles Graber for assistance in the laboratory

Christoph Roth and Gunther Becht for assistance with generating figures for and editing of Chapter 11

James Carr, MD, Dan Gurley, MD, Craig Hansen, MD, Todd Swenning, MD, and Lance Snyder, MD (orthopaedic residents) for their careful review of the developing manuscript and their helpful suggestions

John Osland, MD, for his work in critiquing Chapter 7

David A. McQueen, MD, for his work in critiquing Chapter 11

Danielle Chinn, whose name appropriately appears on the title page, for her superb illustrations, which were done under significant time constraints

Esther Gumpert, Anna Fossella, and Josh Paul of Springer-Verlag, New York, for their patience, understanding, assistance, and faith.

G.L.L.
F.W.C.
E.A.F.

Contents

1

Mechanics

CLINICAL SCENARIO: DISTRACTION FORCE IN TRACTION

Willie Wonderment, 9 years old, was more inquisitive than the typical youngster. Instead of merely wondering if he could jump higher or run faster than the rest of his playmates, he had to prove to himself that he could indeed do so. Not content simply to wonder what was in a bird's nest high in a tree, he climbed up to take a look. Unfortunately, that was his undoing when he

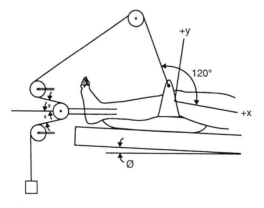

Figure 1.1. Russell's traction, showing how traction is provided at the ankle and support at the knee. A rectangular coordinate system has been positioned with the origin at the axis of rotation at the knee, the positive *x* direction proximal along the axis of the femur and the positive *y* direction anterior. The support force at the knee makes an angle of 120° with the positive *x* axis.

slipped and fell from a limb 15 feet above the ground and sustained a fractured femur. In the hospital emergency room, medical personnel evaluated Willie and, to his parents' relief, found no additional injury. Willie was put to bed on the pediatric ward. Shortly afterward the orthopaedic resident appeared, took off the temporary splint that had been placed on Willie's leg, and set up a skin traction system. This particular traction system, called Russell's traction, is appropriate for a patient of Willie's age, size, and weight and is illustrated in figure 1.1. Treatment of a fracture by traction illustrates several of the laws of mechanics. How can we calculate the amount of weight needed to keep Willie's femur aligned?

In this first chapter we examine several of the laws of mechanics and explore how to use them to answer the question, "How does Russell's traction stabilize Willie's fracture?" We start by defining some terms and presenting some analysis in simple algebraic terms—rather "dry" material, we admit, but working through it will lay a solid foundation for the more interesting, but more complex, orthopaedic biomechanics problems in later chapters.

■ 1.1 MECHANICS

> *Mechanics* is the branch of physics and engineering that deals with forces and the effects produced when forces are applied to objects.

When forces act on an object, the object is changed in some way. The engineering science that deals with forces and their influence on objects is called *mechanics*. An object is any entity that possesses mass, and, in mechanics, such an object is often referred to as a body. This usage should not be confused with the more limited anatomical concept of the corpus humanus.

➤ A *force* is any agency acting on an object that tends to cause it to move, change its motion, or change its size and shape.

Forces are recognized by the effects they produce. If a force is applied to an object or body at rest, it may begin to move; if it is already moving, its motion may be changed. It may speed up, slow down, or change direction. An applied force can also produce a change in a body's size and shape. Forces are usually thought of as pushes or pulls, such as the pull of the traction apparatus on Willie's leg or the pressure of one articulating surface against another in a joint. Other important examples are the frictional forces that act at the surfaces between sliding bodies, the gravitational attraction of the earth's mass that tends to "pull" objects toward its center, and the repulsion, or push, between two magnetic poles of the same sign.

➤ *Dynamics* is the branch of mechanics that deals with the effects that result when forces produce a change in the motion of a body.

➤ *Statics* is the branch of mechanics that deals with the changes in size and shape that are produced when opposing forces are applied to a body but no change in motion occurs.

Mechanics itself is divided into two broad categories, dynamics and statics. *Dynamics* deals with forces that initiate or change the motion of a body, whereas *statics* deals with opposing forces that change a body's size and shape (but not its motion).

■ 1.2 NEWTON'S LAWS

Sir Isaac Newton (1642–1727) is credited with the first correct statement of the laws governing the events that occur when forces are applied to bodies. These statements or laws are the following:

1. If no force is applied to a body, no effect will be produced. As Newton put it, if no force is applied to a body at rest, it will remain at rest, and a body that is moving will continue to move in a straight line at constant velocity. Note that velocity, v, is the distance covered by a moving object in unit time (e.g., meters per second or miles per hour).

2. If a force, F, is applied to a body, the velocity will change; that is, the body will accelerate, and the velocity change, Δv, will be proportional to the force.

$$F \propto \Delta v$$

Because the change in velocity, Δv, is defined as an acceleration, a, we can write

$$F \propto a$$

or

$$F = ma, \tag{1.1}$$

where the proportionality constant, m, is the mass of the body. Equation (1.1) is, of course, Newton's famous second law of motion and describes the relationship between force, mass, and acceleration. Note that the first law is contained within the second law because $a = 0$ (that is, $\Delta v = 0$) when $F = 0$. The field of dynamics is based on Newton's second law.

3. If a force is applied to a body at rest and no acceleration occurs, there must be an equal and opposite force acting on the body. This third law is the basis of statics.

Just because no acceleration results under static conditions, one should not infer that no change of any kind occurs. In fact, when equal and opposite forces act on a body, there is always a change in the shape of the body, which is referred to as deformation. Many of the most interesting and useful problems in orthopaedic biomechanics—such as the forces acting across a joint—are treated using the concepts of statics.

■ 1.3 CHARACTERISTICS OF FORCES

A force is an entity described by two fundamental properties or characteristics: magnitude and direction.

1.3.1 Magnitude

The effect produced when a force acts on a body depends on how large the force is. This property is referred to as the magnitude of the force. In general, the greater the magnitude of a force, the greater will be the effect.

In orthopaedic biomechanics and, in fact, all medical science, the unit of force magnitude is the newton (N). One newton is equal to 0.225 times the weight (force exerted by gravity) of a mass of 1 lb.

$$1 \text{ N} = 0.225 \times 1 \text{ lb (force)}$$

As an example, the force of gravity acting on an apple (i.e., its weight) is about 1 N. How appropriate when we think of the apple dropping on Newton's head!

1.3.2 Direction

The effect produced by a force also depends on the goal or objective toward which the force acts. For example, it is very important whether the muscle forces across a fracture act parallel to the bone axis (producing simple compression) or at an angle to the bone axis (producing bending and angulation at the fracture site).

The concept of direction itself has two elements: *line of action,* which is the line along which a body would move under the influence of the force, and *sense,* or the direction along the line (e.g., left/right, proximal/distal, and so on).

The orientation of the line of action must be expressed by its relation to some convenient frame of reference. For example, in Russell's traction (figure 1.1), the force produced by the sling is said to act along a line originating at the center of the knee and inclined at an angle of 120° anterior to the axis of the femur.

In this figure, a coordinate system is shown with its origin located at the axis of rotation of the knee, the positive *x* direction oriented superiorly along the femoral axis, and the positive *y* direction identical with the anterior direction. Note that the line of action of the force acting through the sling is inclined at an angle φ of 120° from the positive *x* direction. The sense of this force is anterior and slightly inferior.

1.3.3 Vectors

> ➤ A *vector* is a quantity defined by a magnitude and a direction.

The complete quantitative description of many physical entities requires that a single variable, magnitude, be specified. Such single-variable quantities are called *scalars;* time, mass, length, temperature, and heat (caloric content) are examples of scalars. Quantification of certain other entities requires that two variables, magnitude and direction, be specified. These are called *vector quantities.* From the preceeding discussion, it should be clear that force is a vector quantity. Other vectors important in biomechanics are velocity, acceleration, and momentum. Vectors are often represented by a line segment with an arrowhead. The length of the line is proportional to the magnitude of the vector, the orientation of the line segment indicates the vector's line of action, and the arrowhead indicates the sense of the vector along its line of action.

Two additional characteristics of forces are helpful to note: the point of application and the effect produced.

1.3.4 Point of Application

The point of application of a force is the point at which the line of action of a force intersects the surface of the body on which it acts. The insertion of the biceps brachii on the radius is the point of application of the muscle force on the bone, for example.

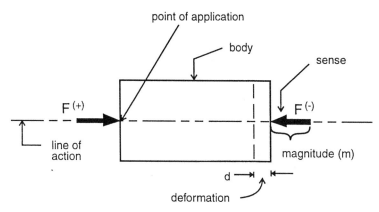

Figure 1.2. Force $F(+)$ and opposing force $F(-)$, both of magnitude m, applied to a body along a common line of action through the point of application to produce a shortening effect, or deformation, d.

1.3.5 Effect

The application of a force to a body produces one of two possible changes: a change in motion (Newton's second law [dynamics]) or a change in shape (Newton's third law [statics]). See figure 1.2 for a pictorial representation of all the characteristics of a force applied to a body under static conditions.

■ 1.4 COORDINATE SYSTEMS

As implied earlier, the location of the coordinate or reference system is actually arbitrary, but a little forethought in picking a convenient location can simplify the subsequent analysis. In orthopaedic biomechanics it is often helpful to relate the coordinate system to the anatomic components under investigation. For example, the center or origin of the coordinate system may be placed at the center of gravity of the whole body, with the positive x axis in the anterior direction, the positive y axis in the left lateral direction, and the positive z axis in the superior direction (figure 1.3a). When a fighter pilot ejects from his or her plane, the ejection force acts in the positive z direction. Similarly, if a single

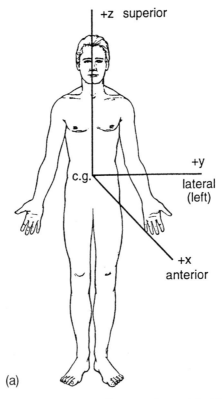

(a)

Figure 1.3. *(a)* Rectangular coordinate system related to the body as a whole. Note the origin is at the center of gravity, $+x$ is anterior, $+y$ is left, and $+z$ is superior. *(b)* Rectangular coordinate system related to the forearm. Note: the origin is at the center of rotation of the elbow, the $+x$ axis coincides with the distal direction along the axis of the lower arm, and the $+y$ axis is in the superior direction. Because a coordinate system was chosen in which all the muscle and gravitational forces act in the x-y plane, this problem has been reduced to a simple two-dimensional analysis.

bone (e.g., ulna) or anatomic unit (e.g., forearm) is being considered, it may be helpful to place the origin at the center of rotation of the relevant joint (e.g., the elbow), with the positive x axis in the distal direction along the axis of the bone or anatomical unit. The positive y axis could then be the superior direction (figure 1.3b). With this choice, all the important muscle and gravity forces are confined to the x-y plane,

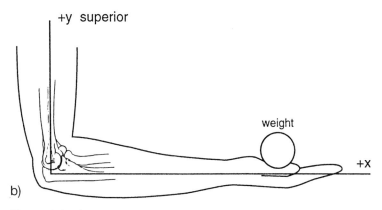

Figure 1.3. (continued)

and the z axis can be ignored, reducing the three-dimensional problem to two dimensions and simplifying the analysis.

■ 1.5 RESOLUTION OF A FORCE INTO ITS COMPONENTS

A directed line segment (arrow) representing a force vector can be drawn on a coordinate system, as shown in figure 1.4. The magnitude is represented by the length of the line segment, and the direction is represented by the angles α, β, and γ the line makes with the positive x, y, and z axes.

This arrangement provides a complete graphical representation of the force vector. The force F can be replaced by three forces, F_x, F_y, and F_z, which are coincident with the $+x$, $+y$, and $+z$ axes and which together produce the same effect as the original force. The original force is called the resultant force, F_R, and the projection of F_R onto the x, y, and z axes comprises its components, F_x, F_y, and F_z (figure 1.5a).

An equivalent result is obtained by placing the component forces head-to-tail starting at the origin, thus bringing the head of the third arrow into exact coincidence with the head of the resultant (figure 1.5b).

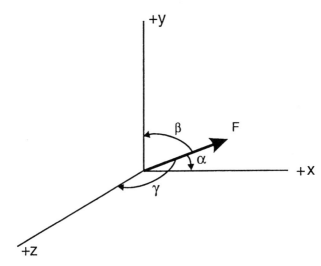

Figure 1.4. Graphical representation of a force vector *(F)* in a three-axis coordinate system where the magnitude of *F* is proportional to the length of the arrow, and the direction is given by the angles (α, β, and γ) between the vector and the *x, y,* and *z* axes. The sense of the direction is given by the arrowhead.

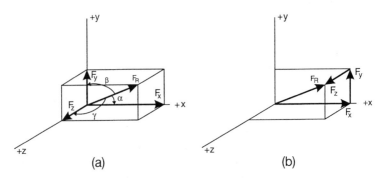

Figure 1.5. *(a)* The resolution of resultant force, F_R, into its components, F_x, F_y, and F_z. *(b)* The head-to-tail arrangement of component forces, F_x, F_y, and F_z, to produce the resultant force, F_R.

■ 1.6 TRIGONOMETRIC ANALYSIS OF FORCE SYSTEMS

The graphical representation of force vectors presented in Section 1.5 is very useful for helping to visualize what is happening, but an exact quantitative analysis by this method requires highly precise and time-consuming drafting procedures. For quantitative results, an analytical approach based on trigonometry is much faster and more accurate. A review of basic trigonometry is presented in figure 1.6 to refresh your memory and help you perform the required calculations.

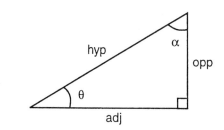

① $\mathrm{Sin}\theta = \dfrac{opp}{hyp}$ ④ $\mathrm{Sin}\alpha = \mathrm{Cos}\theta$

② $\mathrm{Cos}\theta = \dfrac{adj}{hyp}$ ⑤ $opp = hyp\,(\mathrm{Sin}\theta)$

③ $\mathrm{Tan}\theta = \dfrac{opp}{adj}$ ⑥ $adj = hyp\,(\mathrm{Cos}\theta)$

θ	0	15	30	45	60	75	90
Sin θ	0	0.259	0.500	0.707	0.866	0.966	1
Cos θ	1	0.966	0.866	0.707	0.500	0.259	0
Tan θ	0	0.268	0.577	1.00	1.73	3.73	∞

Figure 1.6. Trigonometry refresher.

By trigonometry, then, the magnitude of the components in figure 1.5a can be related to the magnitude of the resultant as follows:

$$F_x = F_R \cos \alpha \tag{1.2}$$

$$F_y = F_R \cos \beta \tag{1.3}$$

$$F_z = F_R \cos \gamma \tag{1.4}$$

■ 1.7 ADDITION OF FORCE VECTORS

One goes to all the trouble of resolving forces into their components for the following reason: The magnitudes of forces can be added only if their vectors are coincident, that is, if they have the same line of action. Thus, in figure 1.7, the magnitudes of F_1 and F_2 cannot be added directly to determine the magnitude of their combined resultant. However, according to the requirement for addition, the magnitudes of the x components, F_{1x} and F_{2x}, can be added because they are coincident.

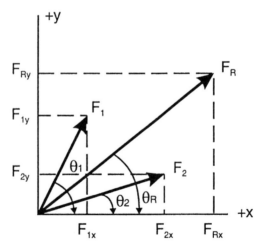

Figure 1.7. Addition of forces F_1 and F_2 in the x-y plane to obtain their combined resultant, F_R. $F_{Rx} = F_{1x} + F_{2x}$ and $F_{Ry} = F_{1y} + F_{2y}$. The magnitude of F_R is $|F_R| = \sqrt{(F_{Rx}^2 + F_{Ry}^2)}$. The direction of F_R is the angle θ_R between F_R and the x axis and can be calculated from $\tan \theta_R = F_{Ry}/F_{Rx}$.

Therefore, the magnitude of the x component of F_R, F_{Rx}, is the sum of F_{1x} and F_{2x}.

$$F_{Rx} = F_{1x} + F_{2x} \tag{1.5}$$

Similarly, the y components can be added to give the y component of F_R.

$$F_{Ry} = F_{1y} + F_{2y} \tag{1.6}$$

The magnitude of the resultant can be obtained from the Pythagorean theorem by the following equation:

$$F_R = \sqrt{F_{Rx}^2 + F_{Ry}^2} \tag{1.7}$$

Finally, the direction of F_R is the angle θ_R, which F_R makes with the x axis. The angle θ_R is given by the following equations:

$$\sin \theta_R = \frac{F_{Ry}}{F_R} \tag{1.8}$$

$$\tan \theta_R = \frac{F_{Ry}}{F_{Rx}} \tag{1.9}$$

For simplicity, force vector addition has just been presented as a two-dimensional problem. Whenever there are only two forces acting through a common point, it is always possible to choose a coordinate system that will reduce the problem to two dimensions. In orthopaedic biomechanics, one always attempts to reduce statics problems to two dimensions, and many important problems have yielded to this approach. For example, one can perform a fairly complete analysis of the forces acting about the knee and the hip by considering only the sagittal plane (knee) or the coronal plane (hip).

If a complete three-dimensional analysis is required, the approach exemplified in figure 1.5 can be generalized to three dimensions. To see this explicitly, the reader is encouraged to write an expression for the magnitude and direction of the resultant force, F_R, that is the equivalent of F_a, F_b, and F_c in figure 1.8.

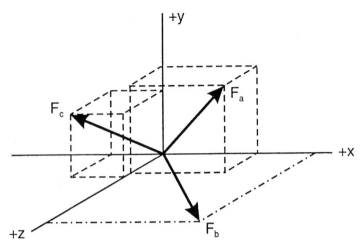

Figure 1.8. Three forces oriented such that F_a lies in the $+x, +y, +z$ quadrant, F_b lies in the $+x, +z$ plane ($F_{by} = 0$), and F_c lies in the $-x, +y, +z$ quadrant. The reader is encouraged to write an expression for the magnitude of F_R in terms of F_{ax}, F_{bx}, F_{cx}, F_{ay}, F_{by}, and so on. In determining the direction of F_R, is the evaluation of a single angle sufficient?

■ 1.8 STATIC EQUILIBRIUM

1.8.1 Two Forces

When a body is at rest (i.e., in a state of static equilibrium) with two forces acting on it, these forces must act along a common line of action and must be of equal magnitude and opposite sense. Furthermore, this arrangement will produce some degree of deformation of the body (see figure 1.2). The possibility that no forces are acting on the body is included by noting that this is just a special case in which the magnitudes of the opposing forces happen to be zero.

1.8.2 Multiple Forces

In the preceding two-force example, the opposing forces were actually added vectorially, and the resulting magnitude was zero, so no movement of the body would occur. This was achieved by simply adding the two magnitudes, one of which was positive and the other, negative. In more complex force systems, it is quite possible to meet the criteria for static equilibrium with three or more noncollinear forces. What is required is that the lines of action of all the forces intersect at a common point. In such a case, the origin of the reference coordinate system should be located at this common intersection point.

As an example of multiple forces acting on a body in static equilibrium, we consider the loading on the patella when the knee is flexed at 90° in a squat or deep knee bend (figure 1.9a). The three major forces acting on the patella are the quadriceps pull, F_Q, the pull of the patellar tendon, F_T, and the reaction force caused by the pressure between the patella and the intercondylar notch, F_C. One should first note that the lines of action of all three forces lie in the sagittal plane and pass through a common point. These are necessary conditions for static equilibrium whenever three or more noncollinear forces act on a body. Forces that do not pass through a common point tend to twist or rotate the body and thus create dynamic conditions.

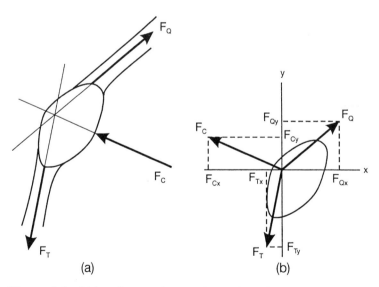

Figure 1.9. *(a)* Loading on the patella produced by the three major forces, quadriceps pull, F_Q, patella tendon pull, F_T, and the reaction (push) against the femoral condyles, F_C. *(b)* A coordinate reference system imposed on the loaded patella showing the x and y components of the three major forces.

This system can next be superimposed on a coordinate system (figure 1.9b), and the components of each force laid out along the x and y axes. The next objective is to determine the direction and magnitude of the one resultant force, F_R, that will produce the same effect as the three applied forces. If this resultant force turns out to have zero magnitude, the conditions for static equilibrium are met.

The x and y components of the resultant, F_{Rx} and F_{Ry}, are found by adding the x components of the applied forces, F_{Qx}, F_{Tx}, and F_{Cx}, to find F_{Rx}, and then by adding F_{Qy}, F_{Ty}, and F_{Cy} to find F_{Ry}. Note that the magnitudes of the x components can be added directly because they are all collinear and the same is true for the y components. In fact, because the patella is in static equilibrium, the components of the applied forces will add up to zero, and the magnitude of the resultant, F_R, is also zero.

$$\Sigma F_x = F_{Rx} = 0 \tag{1.10}$$

$$\Sigma F_y = F_{Ry} = 0 \tag{1.11}$$

$$F_R = \sqrt{F_{Rx}^2 + F_{Ry}^2} = 0 \tag{1.12}$$

1.8.3 Determination of Unknown Forces

The methods of static analysis can help determine the magnitude and direction of an unknown force, which is very useful in biomechanics. For example, a cadaver lower limb can be mounted in a testing fixture and radiographed. It is also relatively easy to attach a clamp to the rectus femoris muscle group and to apply a force of known magnitude to simulate the quadriceps pull (figure 1.9a). As a rough approximation, the patella in the intercondylar notch acts like a pulley, so that one can reasonably assume that the patella tendon pull, F_T, has the same magnitude as F_Q.

The objective now is to find the relationship between F_Q and the force on the patella due to the condyle, F_C. At this point the problem can be greatly simplified by choosing a coordinate system in which the condylar force, F_C, lies along the negative x axis (figure 1.10). From the lateral radiograph, the angular orientation of F_Q and F_T can be estimated, and these angles will be the same; that is, the forces F_Q and F_T are symmetrical about the positive x axis (see angle θ in figure 1.10).

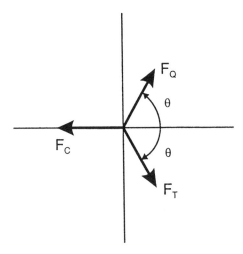

Figure 1.10. Determination of the unknown force between the patella and the condyles, F_C, when the quadriceps force, F_Q, and the patellar tendon pull, F_T, can be estimated.

Only F_Q and F_T have components in the y direction, and, because this is a static case, these y components must be of equal magnitude and opposite direction:

$$F_{Qy} = -F_{Ty}$$

The sum of the components in the x direction can now be written as

$$\Sigma F_x = 0 = F_C + F_{Qx} + F_{Tx}$$

or

$$F_C = -F_Q \cos \theta - F_T \cos \theta.$$

Because F_Q and F_T are equal, we can write

$$F_C = -2F_Q \cos \theta$$

Because θ is approximately half the angle of flexion of the knee, F_C equals approximately $-2F_Q \cos(\phi/2)$, where ϕ is the angle of flexion.

At this point one should ask whether this is a reasonable finding. The answer is yes, at least to the extent that the condylar force, F_C, against the patella will be approximately zero at full extension ($\theta = 90°$), which is to be expected. Furthermore, F_C increases as the angle of knee flexion increases, again as expected.

The determination of F_Q under various circumstances such as walking or stair climbing is also quite feasible. Knowledge of the relationships between the quadriceps pull and the condylar force on the patella can be very useful to a bioengineer designing a patella-resurfacing prosthesis. Finally, one should appreciate that the direct measurement of F_C in a cadaver experiment is difficult because of the slipperiness of the articular cartilage, the curvature of the posterior patellar surface, and the limited room in the intraarticular space.

To conclude this chapter, let us pay a return visit to our patient, Willie, whom we are going to put in Russell's traction. The objective in analyzing the traction system is to determine the relationship between the weights we add to the end of the traction rope, and the magnitude of the distraction force acting across the fracture to maintain the reduction. The first step is to construct a diagram of Willie's leg, showing all the forces acting on it (figure 1.11).

The diagram is somewhat of a simplification in that the leg is shown fully extended with no flexion at the knee. This simplification, however, makes the problem easier to treat at this early stage in the development of our analytical skills.

All the forces acting on the leg are shown, including the traction force, F_t, at the foot; the sling force, F_s, at the knee; the reaction force, F_r, at the hip; the weight of the leg, F_p; and the distributed force along the posterior aspect of the leg (small arrows in figure 1.11), which supports the weight of the leg. A force is assumed to exist at every point where the leg contacts another object (i.e., the distributed force where the leg contacts the mattress and at F_r, where the leg contacts the rest of the body).

Next, the force acting across the fracture is equal to the reaction force, F_r, at the hip because all the traction forces (F_t and F_s) are distal to the fracture (and are opposed by F_r); also, the line of action of F_r is coincident with the axis of the femur. A coordinate system has been chosen in which the force across the fracture lies in the x direction; therefore, only forces in this direction need be considered with regard to distraction of the fracture. None of the forces in the y direction, F_p,

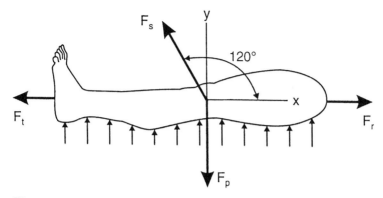

Figure 1.11. A diagram of a leg with a midshaft femoral fracture in a simplified Russell's traction. The simplification consists of showing the knee fully extended so that the traction force at the foot, F_t, is collinear with the femur. This is the principal force maintaining reduction of the fracture. The other forces acting on the leg are the sling force, F_s, acting at the knee; the reaction force, F_r, acting at the hip (i.e., the point of attachment of the leg to the rest of the body); the weight of the leg, F_p; and the distributed force, shown as small arrows along the posterior aspect of the leg. The distributed force provided by contact with the mattress supports the weight of the limb.

the mattress support, and the y component of the sling force (F_{sy}) make any contribution to distraction, although they can lead to angulation of the fracture if not properly balanced. Thus the distraction force at the fracture site is due to only two forces: F_t and the x component of the sling force, F_{sx}. We can therefore write

$$\Sigma F_x = 0 = -F_t - F_s \cos 60° + F_r$$

or

$$F_r = 0.5F_s + F_t. \qquad (1.13)$$

F_s is just the force transmitted by the traction rope and is equal to the weights added. Because the force distracting the fracture, F_{dist}, is equal to F_r, we can further write

$$F_{dist} = 0.5F_{wt} + F_t. \qquad (1.14)$$

All that remains, therefore, is to determine F_t in terms of F_{wt}.

In Russell's traction, the traction force, F_t, is due to the forces transmitted by the ropes through the pulley assembly distal to the foot (figure 1.12a). For the simple arrangement shown in figure 1.12b, the anterior force, F_1, makes an angle θ above the x axis, and the posterior force, F_2, makes an angle θ below the x axis. Of course, the magnitudes of F_1 and F_2 are both equal to the weight, F_{wt}. By inspection, we can conclude that the y components of F_1 and F_2 cancel each other because they are of equal magnitude and opposite direction. The sum of the x components can be written as

$$\Sigma F_x = 0 = -F_1 \cos \theta - F_2 \cos \theta + F_t$$

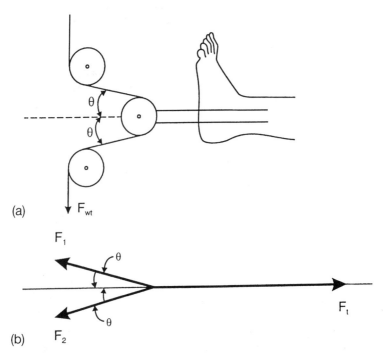

Figure 1.12. (a) The arrangement of the pulleys and traction rope at the foot in Russell's traction. (b) Forces acting at the foot in Russell's traction.

or

$$F_t = F_1 \cos \theta + F_2 \cos \theta.$$

Because F_1 and F_2 both equal F_{wt}, we can write

$$F_t = 2F_{wt} \cos \theta. \qquad (1.15)$$

Substituting this in equation (1.14), we conclude that

$$F_{dist} = 0.5F_{wt} + 2F_{wt} \cos \theta.$$

If θ is small, perhaps 15°, this reduces to

$$F_{dist} = 0.5F_{wt} + 2F_{wt}(0.966)$$

or

$$F_{dist} = 2.4F_{wt} \qquad (1.16)$$

From this we can assume that, in Russell's traction, the force acting to reduce the fracture is about twice the magnitude of the weights added, depending on the angle θ at the foot, the angle of the sling rope at the knee, and frictional losses in the pulleys. Therefore, 5 lb of weights will produce about 10 lb of distraction across Willie's fracture, which should be about right to produce a well-reduced union when healing is complete.

Q1: Clinical Question (Summary)

Willie Wonderment, 9 years old, climbed up a tree to look into the nest and fell about 15 feet to the ground. He fractured his femur and was put to bed on the pediatric ward, where an orthopaedic resident set up a Russell's traction system. How can we calculate the amount of weight needed to keep Willie's femur aligned?

A1: CLINICAL ANSWER

The solution to Willie's traction problem is given in detail in Section 1.8.3. In general, one can assume that, in Russell's traction, the force acting to reduce the fracture is about twice the magnitude of the weights added, depending on the angle θ at the foot, the angle of the sling rope at the knee, and frictional losses in the pulleys. Therefore, 5 lb of weights will produce about 10 lb of distraction across Willie's fracture, which should be about right to produce a well-reduced union when healing is complete. Good thing for Willie that his orthopaedic resident was well versed in biomechanics!

Additional Reading

Ahmed AM, Burke DL, Hyder A: Force analysis of the patellar mechanism. *J Orthop Res* 5:69–85, 1987.

Burstein AM, Wright TM: *Fundamentals of Orthopaedic Biomechanics.* Williams & Wilkins, Baltimore, 1994.

Cochran GVB: *A Primer of Orthopaedic Biomechanics.* Churchill Livingston, New York, 1982.

Meriam JL: *Combined Engineering Mechanics, Statics and Dynamics (SI/English).* John Wiley & Sons, New York 1992.

2

Moments

CLINICAL SCENARIO: FORCES AT THE ELBOW JOINT

A first-year orthopaedic resident, Barkley Brown found himself on radiology service shortly after arriving at Metro General Hospital to start his residency and discovered that he had a little unexpected spare time. Having lifted weights during high school and college to keep in shape for wrestling and football, Dr. Brown welcomed the chance to go to the gym and pump a little iron. He preceded his lifting by doing a series of upper- and lower-body stretches and then started to work on individual muscle groups—first the biceps, then the triceps, then the "pecs," then the "lats," and so on. How much force did he generate across the elbow joint by doing a biceps curl with a 15-kg weight?

In chapter 1, we focused our attention on the effect of forces acting on objects where the lines of action of the forces all passed through a single point. We now expand our analysis to include the situation where the applied forces are of equal magnitude and opposite direction but are parallel, that is, their lines of action do not intersect. This type of loading tends to produce rotation. In figure 2.1, for example, the tangential thrusters on the spacecraft cause it to rotate about its center line. Note that the thrusters do not produce any translation because the upward thrust of one is just canceled by the downward thrust of the other.

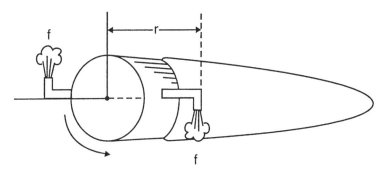

Figure 2.1. Rotation of a spacecraft about its center line as a result of tangential thrusters, each producing a force *f* at a distance *r* from the centerline. The moment *M* produced by this force couple is equal to 2*f* × *r*.

■ 2.1 MOMENTS

The tendency of a force to produce rotation is called a *moment*, and the moment of a given force depends on both the magnitude of the force and the perpendicular distance from the line of action of that force to the axis of rotation. This can be seen in figure 2.2, where the axis of rotation is defined by the door hinges and the distance, *l*, is perpendicular to both the line of action of the force and the axis of rotation. This perpendicular distance is called the *moment arm,* and the magnitude of the moment produced is equal to the product of the force and the length of the moment arm.

$$M = F \times l_{\perp} \qquad (2.1)$$

Note that the units of a moment are force times distance (i.e., newtons times meters, or pounds times inches).

> A moment is the tendency of a force to produce rotation when applied to a body.

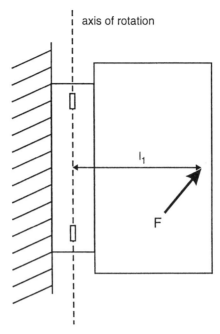

Figure 2.2. The force, F, gives rise to a moment, M, which produces rotation of the door about the axis defined by the hinges. The magnitude of the moment is equal to the product of the force, F, and the moment arm, $l_{\perp}$, which is the perpendicular distance from the axis of rotation to the line of action of the force.

2.1.1 Moments as Vectors

Moments, like forces, are vectors, and, by convention, moments that produce clockwise rotation are considered positive, and those that produce counterclockwise rotation are negative. Moments can be added or subtracted only if they are acting about the same axis of rotation.

The importance of the moment arm is evident if one considers pushing open a heavy door. If one pushes at the middle of the door, the force required is greater than at the edge because the moment arm at the middle is smaller. For this reason, door handles are usually placed as far from the hinge axis as possible.

2.1.2 Couples

> ➤ A couple is a force system consisting of two parallel forces of equal magnitude and opposite direction that produces rotation but no translation.

The thruster forces, f, shown in figure 2.1, produce a couple that causes the spacecraft to rotate, but do not tend to displace it to the side.

■ 2.2 STATICS

When subjected to a moment, an object tends to rotate unless an equal and opposite moment acts on the body. Therefore, we can state that, for static conditions, the sum of the moments about all axes must be zero:

$$\Sigma M_x = 0 \tag{2.2}$$

$$\Sigma M_y = 0 \tag{2.3}$$

$$\Sigma M_z = 0 \tag{2.4}$$

This is in fact an extension of Newton's third law, which we can now state as follows: *If the sum of the forces is zero, there is no translation, and, if the sum of the moments is zero, there is no rotation.*

In the static case, the moments acting on the body deform the body by bending. Thus, in general, we can say that, under static conditions, collinear forces produce tension or compression, and noncolinear parallel forces produce bending. Figure 2.3 shows a simplified diagram of a door with its axis of rotation (hinge axis) in the positive y direction. A force, F_o, is acting to move the door in a counterclockwise direction and is opposed by force F_i, tending to move the door in a clockwise direction. The moment produced by F_o is

$$M_0 = -F_o \times 2l.$$

If the door is in a static equilibrium, the sum of the moments is zero; thus we can write

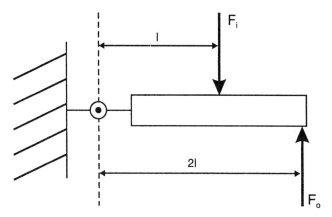

Figure 2.3. A door acted on by two forces (F_i at l and F_o at $2l$) whose moments are of equal magnitude and opposite direction; the door remains stationary (static).

$$\Sigma M_{\text{hinge}} = 0 = - F_o\,(2l) + F_i\,l.$$

Rearranging, we obtain

$$F_i = 2F_o.$$

Thus, the summation of the moments allows us to determine F_i in terms of F_o.

2.2.1 The Free-Body Diagram

We can use the concepts of statics to analyze the effects produced by applied forces and moments, In doing so, we find it helpful to draw a simplified outline diagram of the object under consideration and to indicate the approximate location, direction, and magnitude of all the forces and moments acting on it. Such a simplified drawing is called a *free-body diagram*. A free-body diagram is always limited to a single, rigid, mechanical or structural unit with no flexible joints. Figure 2.4a is a somewhat detailed drawing of Dr. Brown's arm bent 90° at the elbow and holding a 15-kg weight (indicated by P) in his hand. This is *not* a free-body diagram because it is not confined to a single structural unit (it includes a joint), and it does not show all the forces acting on it.

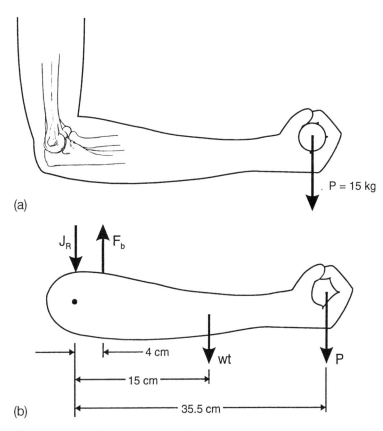

(a)

(b)

Figure 2.4. *(a)* The arm bent at 90° at the elbow, with the wrist and fingers held rigid and a weight of 15 kg held on the palm. *(b)* The free-body diagram of the forearm holding the weight.

Figure 2.4b is a free-body diagram of his forearm, in which the anatomical structures are represented by a simple beam extending from the elbow to the fingers. The wrist, hand, and finger joints are rigidly fixed. All the forces acting on the free body are shown, including the joint reaction force J_R, acting between the ulna and the humerus. Note that in drawing a free-body diagram, it is essential to include a force at every location where the body touches another object because a force may act at any contact point. If, in fact, such a force is zero, it is up to the analyst to show this. The location of all the points of force application on

Dr. Brown's arm can be determined from a radiograph. The force associated with the weight can be measured (P is given as 15 kg), and the weight of the forearm can be assessed from anthropometric data (it is given as 7.5 lb.). This leaves F_b (the biceps force) and J_r as unknowns. It is instructive for Dr. Brown (or any orthopaedic resident) to know how F_b is related to the force of gravity acting on a weight in the hand. Whether in managing an injured elbow or in designing an elbow replacement prosthesis, it is also useful to have an idea of how large the joint reaction force, J_r, is. For these reasons, we attempt to determine F_b and J_r.

First, all units must be converted to SI units (i.e., force in newtons and length in meters):

$$15 \text{ kg} \times 9.806 = 147.1 \text{ N}$$

$$7.5 \text{ lb} \times 4.448 = 33.4 \text{ N}$$

Next, the usual coordinate system is imposed in order to constrain the forearm to move in the x-y plane; the z axis is the axis of rotation of the elbow. Setting the sum of the moments about the elbow equal to zero,

$$\Sigma M_z = 0 = -0.04(F_b) + 0.15(33.4) + 0.355(147.1)$$

and solving for F_b gives

$$F_b = 1{,}430 \text{ N}.$$

Thus the force in the biceps is roughly 10 times that held in the hand. An important technique used in solving this problem was to recognize that the joint reaction force, J_r, creates no moment about the joint axis because its moment arm is zero. Therefore, when the moments were summed about the joint axis, the only unknown force to appear was the biceps force, F_b, which we were able to solve for directly.

Having determined F_b and noting that all the forces are acting in the y direction, we can now solve for J_r by setting the sum of the force in the y direction equal to zero.

$$\Sigma F_y = 0 = -J_r + F_b - \text{wt} - P$$

Substituting and rearranging, we find the following

$$J_r = -1,249.5 \text{ N}$$

Thus, if Dr. Brown is considering going to higher curl weights, he should be interested in knowing that the forces acting across the articulating surface in his elbow will be about 8.5 times greater than the weights in his hand!

■ 2.3 HIP FORCES

By now it should be clear that care in the selection of coordinate systems and in the preparation of free-body diagrams as well as orderliness in the execution of calculations can greatly decrease the burden of biomechanical analyses. Furthermore, the calculations, when completed, can give surprisingly powerful insights into the mechanics of the musculoskeletal system. One of the best examples of this capability can be seen in the analysis of forces acting across the hip. An early treatment of this problem was presented by Victor Frankel, M.D., and Albert Burstein, Ph.D., in their textbook *Orthopaedic Biomechanics,* published in 1970.

The analysis begins with the assumption that the maximum force acting on the head of the femur during the stance phase of gait can be approximated by the static situation of steady one-legged stance. This assumption is generally considered sound because the transition from low loading at the initiation of stance phase to maximum loading at midstance phase occurs relatively slowly, and the intensification of the hip force due to dynamic effects is therefore slight—at least during normal gait. Furthermore, our objective is to develop an overall insight that is valid for the orthopaedic patient population in general. We are therefore forced to forego a detailed analysis of a great many factors (besides loading rate) that can influence the results in a specific case. These additional factors include age, gender, physical condition, pathology, anatomical variations, footwear, and walking surface conditions. Next, we establish a coordinate system with the x axis to the right, the y axis superior, and the z axis anterior and passing through the center of rotation of the femoral head. The z axis serves as the axis of rotation, and we confine our attention to moments acting about this axis (i.e., we consider only abduction and adduction, another important simplifying assumption).

In order to take moments about the hip, we must treat the stance leg and the rest of the body separately. To do this, we construct a free-body diagram of the whole body minus the stance leg (figure 2.5a) and use this to determine the magnitude of the abduction force, F_{ab}, as a function of the body weight, W. From this diagram we can write

$$\Sigma M_C = 0 = -F_{ab}(a) + (5/6)Wb,$$

which reduces to

$$F_{ab} = \frac{5}{6}W\left(\frac{b}{a}\right).$$

Although the ratio b/a varies over a range for different individuals, an acceptable average is 2.4, so that, approximately,

$$F_{ab} = 2W.$$

Next we consider the stance leg as a free body (figure 2.5b). Notice that only anatomic elements important to the solution of the problem are included. We next note that we know the magnitude of the abductor force but not its direction, which we need. From anatomical investigations, we established that the average direction of the abductor muscle fibers relative to the x axis is $60°$. We are now able to determine the x component of the joint force J by summing the forces in the x direction and setting them equal to zero:

$$\Sigma F_x = 0 = F_{ab} \cos 60° - J_x$$

Substituting for F_{ab}, we find that

$$J_x = 1W.$$

We next sum the forces in the y direction and set them equal to zero:

$$\sum F_y = 0 = F_{ab,y} - J_y - \frac{1}{6}W + W$$

Substituting and solving for J_y, we find

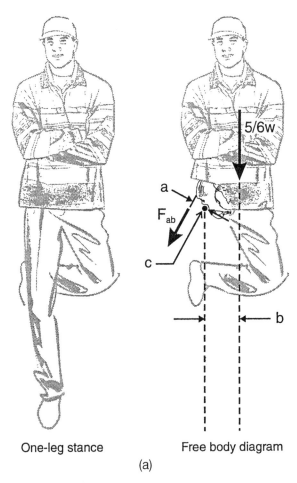

One-leg stance   Free body diagram

(a)

Figure 2.5. *(a)* The free-body diagram of the whole body without the stance leg during one-legged standing. The center of rotation of the hip is point C. Note that the body minus one leg weighs approximately 5/6 of the total body weight, *W*. The line of action of this force does not pass through the normal center of gravity but is shifted toward the non-stance leg because the weight of the stance leg has been excluded from this diagram. *(b)* Free-body diagram of the stance leg showing all the forces acting on it. *Source:* Frankel VH and Burstein AH: *Orthopaedic Biomechanics.* Lea & Febiger, Philadelphia, 1970, pp. 24–25, figures 1.26 and 1.27.

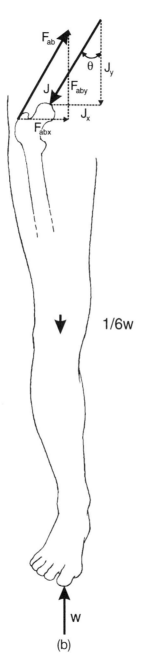

Figure 2.5. (continued)

$$J_y = 2.56\ W$$

We now determine the magnitude of J by the Pythagorean theorem:

$$J = \sqrt{J_x^2 + J_y^2} = 2.75W$$

Thus we find that the force acting on the hip during normal walking is about three times body weight or a little less. This is not a very precise value because of all the assumptions and approximations involved, but it does serve to alert the orthopaedist to the surprisingly large forces that must be managed in such common procedures as a nailed hip fracture or a total hip arthroplasty.

Finally, to complete the analysis, we determine the angle, θ, between the joint force and the y axis. We note that the tangent of θ is

$$\tan \theta = \frac{J_x}{J_y} = \frac{1}{2.56} = 0.391$$

so θ is approximately $20°$ from the y axis (vertical).

Q2: CLINICAL QUESTION (SUMMARY)

Dr. Barkley Brown, a first-year orthopaedic resident, reenergized himself by pumping iron. How much force did he generate across the elbow joint by doing a biceps curl with a 15-kg weight?

A2: CLINICAL ANSWER

The answer to this question can be found in Section 2.2.1, where we determined that Dr. Brown generated about 1,250 N across his elbow joint with each 15-kg biceps curl.

Additional Reading

Burstein AH, Wright TM: *Fundamentals of Orthopaedic Biomechanics.* William and Wilkins, Baltimore, 1994.

Cochran GVB: *A Primer of Orthopaedic Biomechanics.* Churchill Livingston, New York, 1982.

Kyle RF, Wright TM, Burstein AH: Biomechanical analysis of the sliding characteristics of compression hip screws. *J Bone Joint Surg* 62A:1308–1314, 1980.

Meriam JL: *Combined Engineering Mechanics, Statics and Dynamics (SI/ English).* John Wiley & Sons, New York, 1992.

3

Strength of Materials

CLINICAL SCENARIO: COLLES'-TYPE FRACTURE

Fifty-year-old Wilma Jones tripped on the step as she was returning to her apartment and knew immediately—when she put out her hand to break her fall—that she had severely injured her wrist. An X ray confirmed a fracture of the distal radius, Colles' type, and she was treated by a closed manipulation and casting in the emergency room. Why did Wilma's radius break with such a minor fall?

In the first two chapters, we defined forces and moments. In this chapter we examine how forces and moments affect the structure upon which they act. For example, a 10,000-N force applied to one structure may have little effect, whereas a 100-N load applied to a different structure may cause it to shatter. In chapter 3 we explain the concepts of strain and stress. Understanding these fundamental concepts is critical for the future understanding of more advanced principles. We also examine basic static properties of materials with specific application to common orthopaedic biomaterials.

■ 3.1 STRAIN

As discussed in chapter 1, in static equilibrium, forces and moments cause a deformation, or change in shape of a structure. Consider an

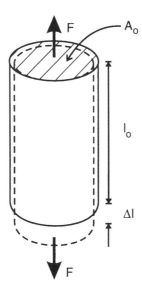

Figure 3.1. An axial force, F, produces deformation, Δl, in this simple cylindrical body. Note that F is distributed over the entire original cross-sectional area, A_o.

axial load, F, applied to a simple cylindrical body with original length l_o and cross-sectional area of A_o, as shown in figure 3.1. The force F will cause a total deformation, or elongation, of the cylinder, which is equal to Δl.

Similarly, it is intuitive that the body will experience twice the deformation, or $2\Delta l$, if twice the load is applied as shown in figure 3.2.

If the force-deformation behavior in these two cases is plotted on a graph, as in figure 3.3, one can see that, for this specimen, the applied force is proportional to the deformation response, or

$$F \propto \Delta l \qquad (3.1)$$

Now, consider further how a force of magnitude F will affect a body of twice the original length ($2l_o$) that has the same cross-sectional area and is made of the same material (figure 3.4). With the same applied load, the body that is twice as long will deform twice as much. Try proving this to yourself by stretching a cut rubber band by gripping it

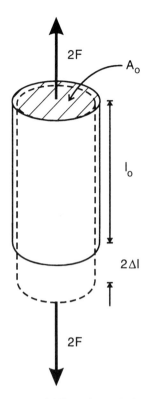

Figure 3.2. An axial force of $2F$ produces twice the deformation in a specimen of the same original length, l_o.

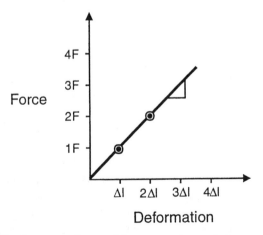

Figure 3.3. For a specimen of the same size and shape and of the same material, the deformation is proportional to the applied load.

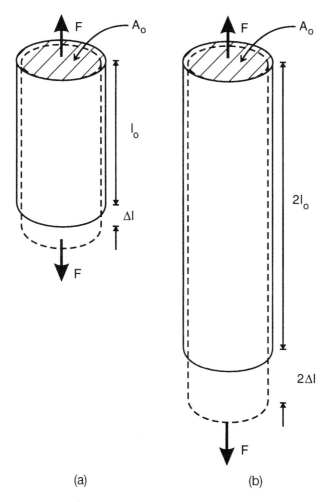

Figure 3.4. With the same applied load, the body that is twice as long will deform twice as much if the original cross-sectional areas, A_o, and material are identical.

in the middle and then at the ends, using approximately the same force each time.

If this new load-deformation response is plotted on the same graph as before (figure 3.5), it is apparent that the slopes of the load-deformation curves for a given material of different lengths are no longer the same.

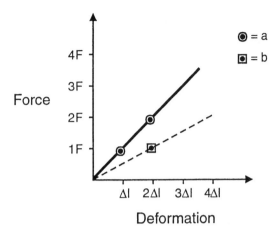

Figure 3.5. For a given force, specimens of the same A_o and the same material will experience different deformations, depending on the length of the specimen. The letter "a" represents data for the specimen of original length l_o; "b" represents data for the specimen of original length $2l_o$.

In order for specimens of varying original lengths to be fairly compared, one must normalize deformation to the original specimen length. Strain is the normalization of deformation to original specimen length and is commonly referred to by the Greek letter ε.

$$\text{Strain} = \varepsilon = \Delta l / l_o$$

So, for the example in figure 3.4, $\varepsilon_a = \Delta l / l_o = 2\Delta l / 2l_o = \varepsilon_b$.

Plotting this new parameter of strain for each of the preceding examples, one can see that force is proportional to strain, regardless of the length of the specimen (see figure 3.6). Both specimens are experiencing the same strain given the same applied load, F.

➢ *Strain* is change in length normalized to the original length.

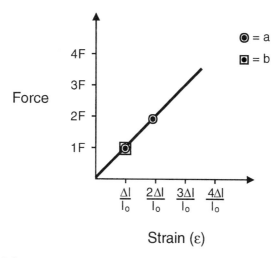

Figure 3.6. For specimens of the same cross-sectional area and material, the applied load is proportional to the strain regardless of original specimen length. The letter "a" represents data for the specimen of original length l_o; "b" represents data for the specimen of original length $2l_o$.

Because length is normalized to length, the units of strain are dimensionless, that is, there are no units. Strain is, however, often reported in terms of millimeters per millimeter or inches per inch. Strain is also noted in terms of the percent strain such that the value of strain is multiplied by 100% and reported in terms of a percentage (for example, 0.1 strain equals 10% strain). One more way in which strain is reported is in terms of microstrain. Often, strain values will be on the order of magnitude of 0.001 strain. Microstrain (or $\mu\varepsilon$) is equal to the value of strain times 10^6 (for example, 0.001 strain = 1,000 $\mu\varepsilon$). We use both percent strain and microstrain values to make the interpretation and presentation of strain values more convenient.

■ 3.2 STRESS

Suppose that one has two specimens of the same material, only now the cross-sectional areas are different; for example, one has twice the original area (figure 3.7). Applying an axial load of force F to each speci-

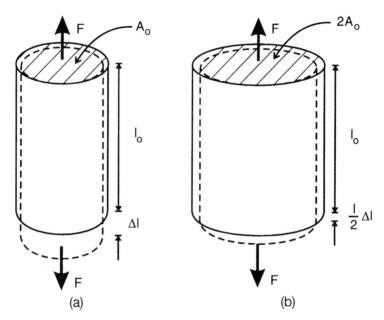

Figure 3.7. A specimen of the same original length and material will deform only one-half as much if the cross-sectional area is doubled.

men, one now finds that the specimen with twice the cross-sectional area experiences only half the deformation of the other specimen.

By plotting this result on the force versus strain curve (figure 3.8), one finds that force is no longer proportional to strain for specimens of the same material and length with different cross-sectional areas. Therefore, in order to characterize a material properly regardless of the size or shape of the specimen, the applied force must be normalized to the original cross-sectional area. Stress is the normalization of applied force to original cross-sectional area and is commonly represented by the Greek letter σ.

$$\text{Stress} = \sigma = F/A_o$$

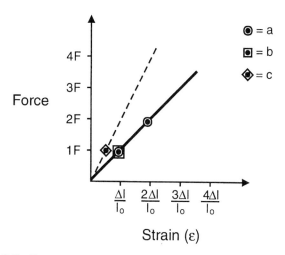

Figure 3.8. Force is no longer proportional to strain for specimens of the same material with different original cross-sectional areas. The letter "a" represents data for the specimen of original length l_o, cross-sectional area A_o; "b" represents data for the specimen of original length $2l_o$, cross-sectional area A_o; "c" represents data for the specimen of original length l_o, cross-sectional area $2A_o$.

Stress is represented by σ and is equal to F/A_o (where A_o is perpendicular to the applied load, F). So, for the example in figures 3.7 and 3.8, $\sigma_a = F/A_{o,a}$, and $\sigma_c = F/A_{o,c} = F/2A_{o,a} = 1/2\ \sigma_a$.

Plotting this new parameter of stress for the previous example, one can now see that, for a given material, stress is proportional to strain, regardless of the cross-sectional area or length of the specimen (see figure 3.9).

By definition, the units of stress are force divided by length squared. In English units, this would be pounds per square inch. In SI units, now the standard for all technical journals, the units of stress are newtons per square meter, or pascals (Pa). To simplify the presentation of stress values for real materials, the units kilopascals (kPa), megapascals (MPa), and gigapascals (GPa) are often employed:

$1\ kPa = 1,000\ Pa$ (for example, $10,000\ Pa = 10\ kPa$)

$1\ MPa = 1 \times 10^6\ Pa$ (for example, $10,000,000\ Pa = 10\ MPa$)

$1\ GPa = 1 \times 10^9\ Pa$ (for example, $1,000,000,000\ Pa = 1\ GPa$)

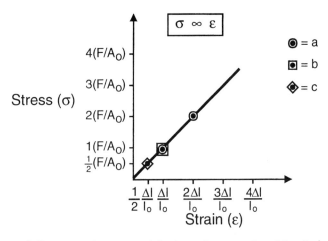

Figure 3.9. For a given material, stress is proportional to strain regardless of the specimen's size and shape. The letter "a" represents data for the specimen of original length l_o, cross-sectional area A_o; "b" represents data for the specimen of original length $2l_o$, cross-sectional area A_o; "c" represents data for the specimen of original length l_o, cross-sectional area $2A_o$.

➤ *Stress* is force normalized to the area over which it is applied.

Most of us understand the quantity of the units of pounds per square inch and what they mean in terms of stress. However, the pascal may be a little less familiar. To grasp the idea of the physical quantity of 1 Pa, one might think of it as the force (or weight) of one medium-sized apple spread out over an average-sized card table. A pascal is a small quantity of stress for most applications; therefore, the terms mega- and gigapascal often come in handy for describing stress values.

Up to this point, only tensile (or pulling) loads have been applied to the specimens. The stresses and strains generated by tensile loading are tensile stress and tensile strain. If compressive (or pushing) loads are applied instead, the same formulas for stress and strain will pertain, but now compressive stresses and compressive strains exist in your structure.

■ 3.3 Stress-Strain Diagram

To summarize the concepts presented in Sections 3.1 and 3.2, the concept of force proportional to deformation cannot be used to compare specimens of different sizes and shapes of even the same material. By normalizing force and deformation to stress and strain, comparisons of various *materials* can now be made, regardless of the specimen size and shape. In other words,

$$\sigma \propto \varepsilon$$

for a given material in the linear elastic region.

If this relationship is plotted on a graph (figure 3.10), one can see that the slope of the line relates the stress and strain. Remember from algebra that a straight line can be modeled by the equation

$$y = mx + b,$$

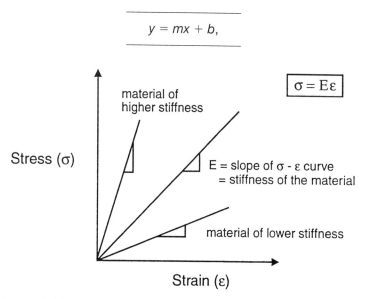

Figure 3.10. Generic σ-ε curve (linear elastic region only) for materials of various stiffness.

where m is the slope and b is the y intercept. Using this relationship to model linear elastic material behavior, one sees that the stress can be related to the strain as

$$\sigma = E\varepsilon + 0 \quad \text{or} \quad \sigma = E\varepsilon$$

This relationship is commonly referred to as Hooke's Law, named after the man who first explained it. The factor E is referred to by a variety of different names such as the proportionality constant, elastic modulus, modulus of elasticity, or Young's modulus. A constant value for a specific linear elastic material, E is a property of the material and is not dependent on the size and shape of the specimen.

> ➤ One name for the stiffness of a material is *Young's modulus,* named for Thomas Young, whose first formal studies were in medicine. He received his doctor's degree in medicine in 1796 and later applied his genius to solving problems in the physical sciences and mechanics.

■ 3.4 MODULUS OF ELASTICITY (OR YOUNG'S MODULUS)

The modulus of elasticity of a material, E, is the material property that relates stress to strain. E is used to describe how stiff a material is in tension and compression. E is independent of the size and shape of the specimen.

A linear elastic material can be modeled as a spring (figure 3.11). The relationship $F = Ku$ describes the deformation, u, that a spring of spring stiffness K experiences when pulled with force F. Just as a spring recovers all the deformation applied when the force F is taken away, so a linear elastic material returns to its original shape when an externally applied stress is removed.

Just as different springs have different stiffnesses, different materials have different elastic moduli. For example, we all recognize that the

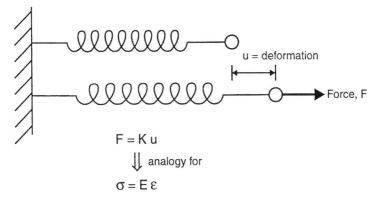

Figure 3.11. The linear elastic region of material behavior can be thought of as a spring whose deformation is completely recoverable within the limits of the spring.

material from which a rubber band is made will stretch much further than a metal paper clip with about the same cross-sectional area. The same is true when comparing various metals. Even though one cannot detect a difference in the way metals behave by pulling them in one's bare hands, special techniques exist (see chapter 12) that allow measurement of slight, but often very important, differences in stiffnesses of materials.

3.4.1 Elastic Moduli of Some Common Orthopaedic Materials

The elastic modulus or stiffness of orthopaedic materials is an important factor in determining the response of the material in a structure and in design. For example, stainless steel is about twice as stiff as pure titanium. For that reason, some manufacturers promote the use of titanium bone plates to reduce the effect of stress shielding on bone. A list of some common orthopaedic biomaterials and their approximate elastic moduli is presented in table 3.1. An easy way to remember the elastic moduli of these materials is by using the rule of ones and twos. Rounding the elastic moduli up or down, as shown in table 3.1, allows for easy recollection of the approximate stiffness values. Of course, these values should never be used in design, but they come in handy when reading medical literature, listening to implant company repre-

Table 3.1   Approximate elastic moduli of some common orthopedic biomaterials

Orthopaedic biomaterial	Approximate elastic modulus (GPa)	Modulus by rule of ones and twos (GPa)
Co-Cr alloys	210	200
Stainless steel, 316	190	200
Titanium implant alloy (Ti-6Al-4V)	110	100
Cortical bone	12–24[a]	20
PMMA bone cement	2.2	2
Ultrahigh molecular weight polyethylene (UHMWPE)	1.2	1
Cancellous bone	0.005–1.5[a]	0.01–2

[a] Depends strongly on density and/or direction

sentatives, and answering Orthopaedic In-Training Examination (OITE) or board questions.

■ 3.5 STRENGTH AND OTHER MATERIAL PROPERTIES FROM THE STRESS-STRAIN CURVE

So far, only the linear elastic region of the stress-strain curve has been examined. However, from simply bending a paper clip, one can clearly see that not all deformation is recoverable. Some materials can be deformed past the elastic limit, and at least part of the deformation remains after the load is removed. This type of deformation is called *plastic deformation*. Almost all metals and most other materials exhibit some degree of plastic deformation.

On a stress-strain curve, plastic deformation appears as a nonlinearity (figure 3.12). In the nonlinear portion of the stress-strain curve, Hooke's law ($\sigma = E\varepsilon$) no longer applies. Many material properties other than the elastic modulus can be obtained from the stress-strain curve taken beyond elastic behavior to fracture.

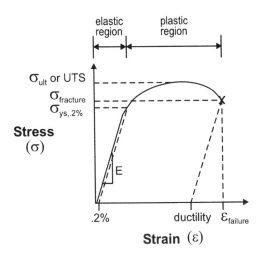

E : modulus of elasticity
    (or elastic modulus or Young's modulus)

$\sigma_{ys,.2\%}$: 0.2% offset yield strength

$\sigma_{fracture}$: fracture strength (or stress at fracture)

σ_{ult} or UTS : ultimate tensile strength (or highest stress reached)

toughness : area under the $\sigma-\varepsilon$ curve (or work to failure)

$\varepsilon_{failure}$: strain at fracture

ductility : plastic strain at failure

Figure 3.12. Typical σ-ε curve for a material that exhibits plastic deformation.

Stress values that are critical in defining material behavior are referred to as strength values. *Yield strength* (σ_{yield}) is the stress at which plastic deformation begins. The *ultimate tensile strength* (σ_{ULT}, or UTS) is the maximum stress a material can undergo before failure or breakage of the material is imminent. The *fracture strength* (which is sometimes equal to the UTS) is the stress at which fracture actually occurs. These strength parameters are used in engineering design of structures to predict when failure will occur.

Other material properties that can be obtained from the σ versus ε curve are *strain at fracture*, the *ductility* of the material (or the amount of plastic strain a material can store before failure), the *toughness* of the material, and, of course, the elastic modulus. In subsequent chapters we will discuss all of these parameters further.

3.5.1 Strength and Stiffness of Bone: Cortical Versus Cancellous

In table 3.1, a range of elastic modulus values (which are dependent upon the density and direction in which the modulus is measured) were given for cancellous and cortical bone. Materials that have the same properties in all directions are referred to as *isotropic;* materials that display different material properties in different directions are called *anisotropic.* Bone is anisotropic, as is almost every biological tissue.

The strength of bone is dependent on its density and structure and the direction in which strength is measured. Osteoporotic bone (which has reduced density) is much weaker than normal, healthy bone. Even in normal, healthy bone, the structure of haversian bone leads to an inherently anisotropic material; the strength of the bone transverse to the osteonal structure is less than in the direction of the osteons. Cancellous bone is formed not only in a variety of different basic structures but can also be found in densities ranging from nearly solid to mostly porous. Many more details on the subjects of tissue structure, strength, and function will be covered in chapters 6, 9, and 17.

■ 3.6 SHEAR STRESS, STRAIN, AND MODULUS

Take a stack of loose papers and try pushing flat across the top of the stack. The sheets of paper move past each other in shear because of the shear force you applied. By definition, a force applied in line with a surface is a *shear force.* The movement of the top sheet of paper from its original position is the deformation caused by the applied shear force. The concepts of shear force and deformation are illustrated in figure 3.13. Analysis of stresses and strains resulting from a shear force is similar to the case of the axial force, except that, in the calculation of *shear stress,* the area over which the force acts is parallel to the applied force. *Shear strain* is calculated from the deformation normalized to the original height of the specimen perpendicular to the deformation. Shear stress, τ, and shear strain, γ, can then be defined as

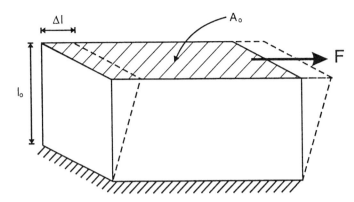

Figure 3.13. A shear force, F, produces deformation, Δl, in this simple rectangular body. Note that F is distributed over the entire original cross-sectional area, A_o, parallel to F and Δl's perpendicular to l_o.

$$\text{shear stress} = \tau = F/A_{o\|},$$

where $A_{o\|}$ is parallel to the applied load, F, and

$$\text{shear strain} = \gamma = \Delta l / l_{o\perp},$$

where $l_{o\perp}$ is perpendicular to the deformation, Δl.

➢ Shear stress is the stress produced when a force acts in line with a surface. Shear stress (τ) is related to shear strain (γ) by the shear modulus *(G)*.

Shear stress and shear strain are proportional for a given material in the elastic range. The shear modulus (usually referred to as G) is the parameter that relates shear stress to shear strain; the shear modulus of a material indicates how stiff it is in shear. The relationship of shear stress to shear strain has the same form as that for tensile (and compressive) stress and strain where

$$\tau = G\gamma$$

For most materials, the shear modulus is about one-half to one-third of the elastic modulus.

Q3: CLINICAL QUESTION (SUMMARY)

Wilma tripped on a step and broke her fall (and her wrist!). The X ray showed a Colles'-type fracture. Why did Wilma's radius break with such a minor fall?

A3: CLINICAL ANSWER

Colles' fracture is the most common type of fracture that occurs when a person trips and tries to break his or her fall with an out-stretched hand. When trying to reproduce this type of fracture in the laboratory, investigators found that the most reliable wrist and loading position was 70° to 80° of dorsiflexion and 5° of radial deviation with the impact force aligned with the long axis of the radius. This type of impact usually creates a transverse fracture in the distal metaphysis of the radius as a result of compressive failure of the cancellous metaphyseal bone. As will be discussed briefly in Section 9.1, bone is weakest in shear and will usually fail in a shear mode when subjected to compressive loading. We discuss the strength of tissues and failure modes of bone further in chapters 9 and 17.

Additional Reading

Black J: *Orthopaedic Biomaterials in Research and Practice.* Churchill Livingstone, New York, 1988.

Cochran GVB: *A Primer of Orthopaedic Biomechanics.* Churchill Livingstone, New York, 1982.

Hayes WC: Biomechanics of cortical and trabecular bone: Implications for assessment of fracture risk. In *Basic Orthopaedic Biomechanics,* VC Mow, WC Hayes, Eds. Raven Press, New York, 1991.

Orthopaedic Science: A Resource and Self-Study Guide for the Practitioner. American Academy of Orthopaedic Surgeons, Park Ridge, Ill., 1986 (ISBN O-89203-011-9).

4

Stresses in Bending

CLINICAL SCENARIO: FRACTURE OF THE FEMORAL NECK

Mabel Able, 80 years old, lived alone in a two-story house taking care of her own needs, such as cooking, cleaning, and tending a small garden and a flower bed. Until about two years ago she also walked around the block every day but recently has confined her-

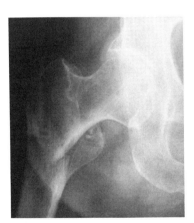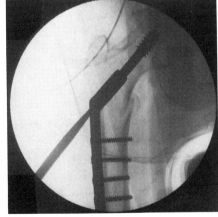

Figure 4.1. Pre- and intra-operative radiographs of a fractured proximal femur.

self to her house and yard. Her next-door neighbor comes by to check on her every day and helps her with her grocery list, mails packages for her, and so on. On Monday morning when the neighbor went to check Mabel, she found Mabel lying on the kitchen floor, moaning and complaining of pain in her right hip. The neighbor could see that the leg was turned out and shortened, and she immediately suspected that Mabel had slipped on the linoleum when she came downstairs to make her morning coffee. The rescue squad was called, and Mabel was transported to the hospital, where the suspicion of a fractured hip was confirmed by a radiograph. After her family doctor came in and pronounced Mabel fit for surgery, she was taken to the operating room, where internal fixation with a compression screw and side plate was accomplished without any complications. The pre- and intra-operative X rays are shown in figure 4.1. What were the mechanical factors causing Mabel's hip to break?

In chapter 3, the basic concepts of stress and strain were introduced by examining the effects of axial, tensile, and compressive loads on structures of known cross-sectional areas. In real life, however, very few structures are subjected to pure tension or compression. In the human body, bending is the predominant form of loading of bones and implants. In this chapter, you will take a moment to learn what kinds of stresses are generated in bending and how to estimate failure of structures in bending.

■ 4.1 STRESSES IN BENDING

Consider a beam that is attached at one end and free at the other. If a force is applied at the free end at the posterior side (figure 4.2a), the beam will bend anteriorly in the direction of the force. The bending moment produced by the applied force causes the material in the deformed beam to be stretched apart (or put in tension) on the posterior side and pushed together (or compressed) on the anterior side. Therefore, the beam experiences tensile stresses on the posterior side and compressive stresses on the anterior side. Compare this beam (com-

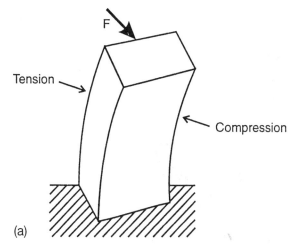

(a)

Figure 4.2. *(a)* A beam that is subjected to bending will experience tension on one side and compression on the other. This situation is similar to flexion and extension bending of the spinal column. In flexion *(b)*, the anterior side is compressed, and the posterior side is spread apart. In extension *(c)*, anterior side is spread apart and the posterior side is compressed.

monly called a cantilever beam) and loading with the spinal column in figure 4.2b. Just as with the beam, under normal forward bending (or flexion), the spinal column experiences tension on the posterior side and compression on the anterior side.

Through any given horizontal section of the beam, there is a gradation of stresses from highest tensile on the posterior edge to highest compressive on the anterior edge. Figure 4.3 shows a closer look at a section of the beam from figure 4.2a. The gradation of stress in the section is linear, with zero stress at the midpoint line of the symmetric section. This line of zero stress is called the neutral axis; the neutral axis represents the axis about which rotation of the beam section would take place if no constraints were applied. In a symmetric section, the neutral axis splits the section into two identical halves; in an asymmetric section (such as a triangular section), the location of the neutral axis can be precisely calculated without much trouble, but as a quick rule of thumb, it separates the area of the section into two approximately equal halves.

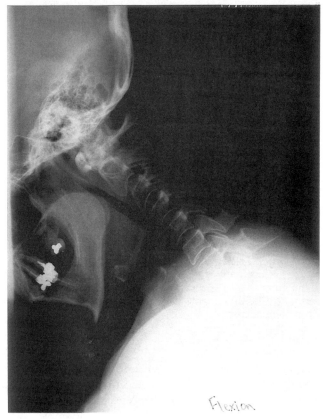

(b)

Figure 4.2. (continued)

> ➢ The *neutral axis* is the axis of zero stress that
>   separates tension and compression in a
>   structure under bending. It would be the
>   axis about which rotation would occur if the
>   structure were not constrained.

Clearly, the stresses at the posterior edge of the beam (figure 4.2a)
are not the same along the entire length of the beam. Even though the

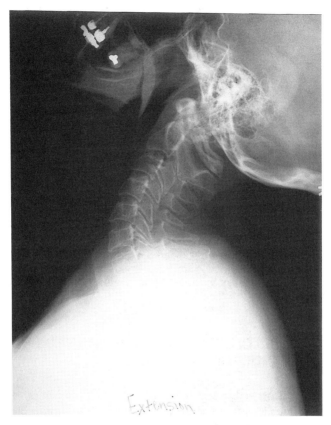

(c)

Figure 4.2. (continued)

beam displacement through space is the greatest at the top, or free, end of the beam, the material there is being stretched the least and experiences the lowest stress and strain. Likewise, the material near the fixed end of the beam is displaced the least but experiences the greatest amount of material deformation and tensile stress.

Prove these ideas to yourself by making equally spaced grid marks on the edges of an eraser. Bend it at one end, and watch the spaces grow or shrink along the length and through the section of the eraser.

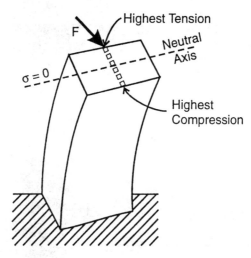

Figure 4.3. A structure subjected to bending exhibits a gradation of stresses across a section from maximum tension on the outer edge through zero stress at the neutral axis to maximum compression on the inner edge.

■ 4.2 CALCULATING STRESSES DUE TO BENDING IN STRUCTURES

Stresses generated in structures during bending are directly related to the magnitude of the bending moment applied. In the previous case of the beam in cantilever bending, the greatest stress occurred where the moment was maximum: at the fixed end of the beam.

The equation relating bending stress to bending moment is:

$$\sigma = \frac{My}{I} \quad \text{STRESSES IN BENDING} \qquad (4.1)$$

where σ = stress

M = applied moment at a given point along the beam

y = distance from neutral axis to the point where stress is to be calculated

I = section shape parameter known as the area
moment of inertia or the second moment of
inertia

From this equation, one can see that stress is directly proportional to
the moment applied to the section. In addition, if the location in the section where one wants to calculate stress is right at the neutral axis, then
$y = 0$, and the stress is equal to zero. This concurs with the basic concept of the neutral axis being the axis of zero stress.

The final parameter in the equation for calculating stresses in bending is I, the area moment of inertia. The area moment of inertia (I) is a
quantifiable parameter that reveals why some shapes are more rigid
than others. It is related to the spatial distribution of material in relation
to the neutral axis: The farther away the material from the neutral axis,
the greater the structure's resistance to bending. The units of I are
length to the fourth power.

➢ The *area moment of inertia (I)* is a quantifiable parameter that describes the spatial
distribution of the material in a structure
section in relation to its neutral axis. *I* is a
sectional property of the structure and is not
related to the type of material from which
the structure is made.

To understand this concept better, consider how one can bend a con-
crete reinforcing rod, $\frac{3}{8}$ inch in diameter, in comparison to a metal pipe
used for plumbing, shown schematically in figures 4.4a and 4.4b. In
this example, the rod and pipe are made of similar materials and have
identical cross-sectional areas, A_0. Intuitively one knows that it is much
easier to bend the rod than the pipe. Why is this so? The rod has a much
lower area moment of inertia (I) than the pipe and is therefore less resistant to bending forces and moments.

Again prove this concept to yourself by bending a common plastic
ruler along its length, first in the most flexible orientation and then at
90°. Determine where the ruler section's neutral axis is in each orienta-

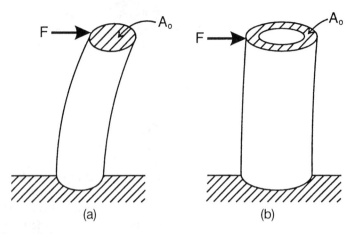

(a)   (b)

Figure 4.4. Two steel cylindrical structures, one, a solid rod *(a)*, and the other, a pipe *(b)*, are subjected to the same bending moment. The pipe deforms less than the rod because it has a larger area moment of inertia.

tion; remember that the neutral axis splits tension and compression. Explain why the second orientation is so much more rigid than the first in terms of the neutral axis and the area moment of inertia.

■ 4.3 DETERMINING AREA MOMENT OF INERTIA *(I)*

Figure 4.5 lists the formulas for area moments of inertia for several common shapes. *It is not important for you to memorize or remember the exact formula for each shape.* Rather, it is important to remember three basic concepts:

1. In a rectangular cross-section structure, the distance perpendicular to the neutral axis has a third-power effect on I

2. In a circular-section structure, the radius has a fourth-power effect on I

3. For hollow sections symmetric about the neutral axis (such as a pipe), the net I value is equal to the I of the outer section minus the I of the missing inner section.

Shape	Area Moment of Inertia I
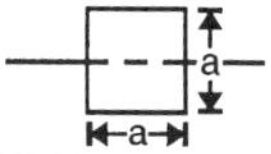	$\dfrac{1}{12}\,a^4$
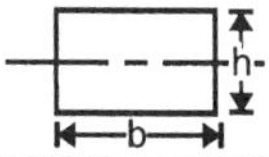	$\dfrac{1}{12}\,bh^3$
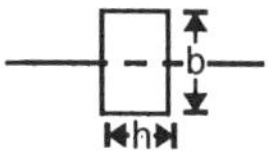	$\dfrac{1}{12}\,hb^3$
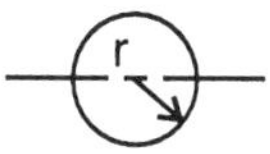	$\dfrac{\pi}{4}\,r^4$
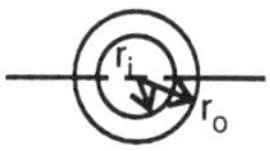	$\dfrac{\pi}{4}\,(r_o^4 - r_i^4)$

Figure 4.5. Formulas to calculate the area moment of inertia for several common cross-section shapes.

From the rectangular shapes shown in figure 4.5, please note that the specific symbols used for distance along and away from the neutral axis have no meaning. If b and h are equal for these two orientations, the second rectangle, turned 90° from the first, has a much greater I value because it has more material distributed far away from the neutral axis.

■ **4.4 DETERMINING STRESSES IN REAL STRUCTURES**

As stated in equation 4.1, stresses in structures undergoing bending are a function of the moment and structural geometry. To restate, the equation for determining stresses in bending of structures composed of one material is:

$$\sigma = \frac{My}{I} \quad \text{STRESSES IN BENDING} \quad (4.1)$$

It is important to note that stresses in bending depend only on the applied forces and size and shape of the structure, *not on the material* from which it is manufactured. For example, an intramedullary rod made out of a cheap plastic and another made from stainless steel experience the same stress under identical loading conditions. However, the steel rod would obviously withstand much higher loads before it broke and would work much better for fracture fixation by allowing less deformation.

Some examples of the use of this equation in orthopaedics are as follows.

Example: Stress at the Neck of a Femoral Implant

The neck region in the femoral component of total hip implants can be a critical region of design.

1. How much stress does the base of the neck of a typical implant (figure 4.6) experience during the stance phase of gait?

2. Will the neck of the femoral implant ever fracture? (The implant material is a typical cobalt-chromium (CoCr) alloy. Assume UTS = 800 MPa and endurance limit 350 MPa [endurance limit is the stress at which the material will not break even under repeated cyclic loading].)

3. What would be the stress at the neck region if the implant were made out of a plastic material, $E = 2.0$ GPa?

Assume two-dimensional loading as shown in figure 4.6, with the load acting through the center of the femoral head.

Solution: The stress at the base of the neck is equal to My/I, as stated in equation 4.1. In this example,

$$M = P \times \text{moment arm} = 2{,}400 \text{ N} \times 18 \text{ mm}$$
$$= 43{,}200 \text{ N mm} = 43.2 \text{ N m}$$

$$y = r = 6.5 \text{ mm} = 0.0065 \text{ m}$$

$$I = \frac{\pi}{4}r^4 = (3.14/4)(0.0065 \text{ m})^4 = 1.4 \times 10^{-9} \text{ m}^4$$

$$\sigma_{\text{stance}} = \frac{My}{I} = \frac{(43.2 \text{ N m})(0.0065 \text{ m})}{(1.4 \times 10^{-9} \text{ m}^4)}$$
$$= 200 \times 10^6 \text{ N/m}^2 = 200 \text{ MPa}.$$

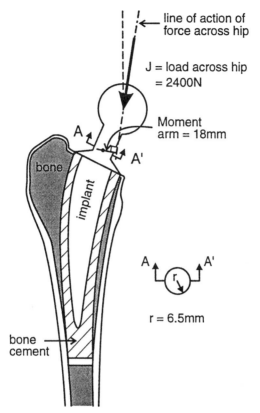

Figure 4.6. A total hip femoral component is subjected to bending. The maximum tensile stress at the taper region in one-legged stance is estimated to be about 200 MPa.

Therefore, the neck of the cobalt-chromium (CoCr) alloy femoral implant should not fracture during normal one-legged stance because the stress at the tension side of the neck is less than the ultimate tensile stress and the endurance limit of the material (see chapters 8 and 11 for further explanation of the endurance limit). If the neck did fracture at this region, many other factors may be responsible. (These ideas are also explored in chapters 8 and 11.)

If the implant were composed of a plastic material ($E = 2.0$ GPa), the stress at the neck region would still be 200 MPa under single-leg stance. The stress in a structure is not dependent on the material from which it is made. Because the UTS of most plastics is often well below

200 MPa, however, the plastic implant would probably break the first time the patient was fully weight-bearing.

■ 4.5 BENDING RIGIDITY

By definition, a structure's bending rigidity is its ability to resist bending deformation. The more rigid a structure, the less it bends under a given load. Although the stress is the same in beams of identical cross-sectional shapes made from steel and rubber, it is obvious that the rubber beam will deform more than the steel beam. Rigidity of a section of a structure made from one material is defined by the factor EI (modulus of elasticity multiplied by the area moment of inertia of the section). Therefore, if two devices are of the same shape, but one is made from a cobalt-chromium alloy and the other, from a titanium alloy, the former device will be about twice as rigid as the latter. Similarly, a doubling of the thickness of a bone plate (figure 4.7) will increase the rigidity of the plate by a factor of 2^3, or 8. This is determined by

$$\frac{\text{Rigidity}_{\text{2t plate}}}{\text{Rigidity}_{\text{1t plate}}} = \frac{E_{\text{2t plate}} I_{\text{2t plate}}}{E_{\text{1t plate}} I_{\text{1t plate}}} = \frac{I_{\text{2t plate}}}{I_{\text{1t plate}}}$$

$$= \frac{\frac{1}{12}(b)(h_{\text{2t plate}})^3}{\frac{1}{12}(b)(h_{\text{1t plate}})^3} = \frac{(h_{\text{2t plate}})^3}{(h_{\text{1t plate}})^3} = \left[\frac{h_{\text{2t plate}}}{h_{\text{1t plate}}}\right]^3 = 2^3.$$

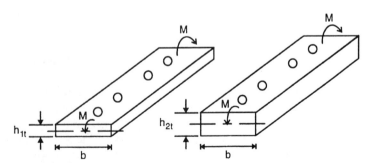

Figure 4.7. Doubling the thickness of a bone plate will increase its bending rigidity by a factor of 8.

Q4: Clinical Question (Summary)

Mabel Able appeared to have slipped and broken her femoral neck after two years of limited activity. What were the mechanical factors causing Mabel's hip to break?

A4: Clinical Answer

Mabel's hip probably broke due to the bending moment applied to it during the fall. However, that is not the whole answer to this puzzle. Mabel may have been experiencing a gradual reduction in her bone quality and strength (osteoporosis), not unusual in an 80-year-old woman. It is possible that Mabel had been developing progressive damage to her hip in the form of fatigue (or stress) fractures— little cracks that do not cause immediate failure and may heal naturally in a younger person— but that for Mabel eventually added up to a weakened hip that could easily break with a slight overload. These little cracks may have caused her some pain with walking, which might have led to her recent reduction in activity. It is even possible that Mabel did not actually slip but only appeared to do so because her femur had finally completed fracture, and her leg gave way!

The next puzzle is, why did her fracture occur at the femoral neck and not at a different location on the femur? The answer to this is that the greatest stress (combined with the weaker material) occurred at the femoral neck. Even in bones that have not experienced the effects of osteoporosis, the femur will break at the femoral neck under excessive axial loading.

Further Reading

Beer FP, Johnston ER: *Mechanics of Materials.* McGraw-Hill, New York, 1981.

Burstein AH, Wright TM: *Fundamentals of Orthopaedic Biomechanics.* Williams & Wilkins, Baltimore, 1994.

Hayes WC: Biomechanics of cortical and trabecular bone: Implications for assessment of fracture risk. In *Basic Orthopaedic Biomechanics,* VC Mow, WC Hayes, Eds. Raven Press, New York, pp. 93–142, 1991.

Huiskes R: Principles and methods of solid biomechanics. In *Functional Behavior of Orthopedic Biomaterials,* P Ducheyne, GW Hastings, Eds. CRC Press, Boca Raton, pp. 51–98, 1984.

Orthopaedic Science: A Resource and Self-Study Guide for the Practitioner. American Academy of Orthopaedic Surgeons, Park Ridge, Ill., 1986 (ISBN O-89203-011-9).

5

Stresses in Torsion

CLINICAL SCENARIO: SPIRAL FRACTURE OF THE TIBIA WHILE SKIING

Sandra Snowflake, an X-ray technician at Mega General Hospital, spent most of her spare time either in the gym or in the park running. Thus she was in excellent physical shape. Her major reason for staying in shape was her love of skiing, and she worked and lived for the three separate weeks she took for ski vacations in Colorado. This year spring skiing was exceptionally good, and she was at the top of her form, schussing down the black diamond runs with ease. Unfortunately, the new bindings she was getting used to had not been adjusted exactly right, and she knew immediately—when she hit the icy patch and lost control of her outside ski—that her leg was broken. This was confirmed at the small hospital at the base of the slope where she was taken by the ski patrol. When Dr. Fromm showed her the film of her leg, her experienced eye recognized a spiral fracture of the tibia. Why does torsion create a tibial fracture?

In the previous chapter, the basic concepts of stresses in bending were introduced. In this chapter, we take a couple of moments to look at stresses generated from applied torques. Torque is a moment that produces spinning in an unconstrained body and twisting deformation in a constrained body. Many parts of the human body (for example, the proximal femur and the ankle) experience significant torque during normal activities. In this chapter we examine stresses generated from torques and see why spiral fractures occur in bone loaded to failure in torsion.

■ 5.1 STRESSES IN TORSION

Consider two equal and opposite forces applied to a cylinder (figure 5.1). If the cylinder is not constrained, application of these two forces will cause it to spin. When the object is constrained in space, the two forces, by definition, form a couple, or a pure torque, that twists the cylinder. A torque is a moment that produces twisting in a structure. In the example in figure 5.1, the two forces, F, times their moment arm, r, produce a torque, T.

Shear stresses are generated in structures when torque is applied as shown in figure 5.2. In this figure, a tiny cube of material from the

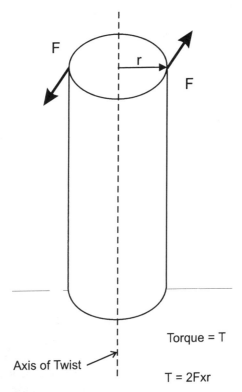

Torque = T

Axis of Twist

T = 2Fxr

Figure 5.1. A pure torque is created by two forces acting as a couple about an axis of twist. If the object is not constrained, it will spin in space.

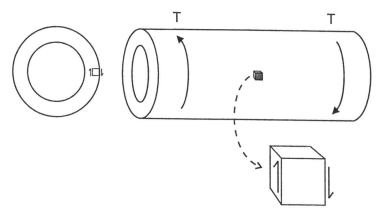

Figure 5.2. Shear stresses are generated from applied torques. The two shear forces shown in the picture are not the only forces acting on the cube. What would happen to the cube if there were not additional shear forces acting on the top and bottom faces?

cylinder is depicted to show the shear acting as a result of the applied torque. Through any given horizontal cross section of the cylinder, there is a gradation of shear stresses from highest at the outer edge to zero at the center point. The axis of the center points of all the cross sections is called the axis of twist; it is the line of zero stress in structures in pure torsion.

➢ The *axis of twist* is the line or axis of zero stress in the center of an axisymmetric structure at which the stress is zero when the structure is subjected to torsional loading. It is the axis about which the object would spin if not constrained.

In a cylinder subjected to pure torque, the shear stress and shear strain on the outer surface are equal along the length of the cylinder. Even though the fixed end of the cylinder does not move through space, it experiences the same shear stress and strain as the rest of the structure. Prove this to yourself by marking small same-size squares along the length of a cylindrical rubber eraser (like the kind used in mechanical pencils). As you twist the eraser, the squares become identical parallelograms along the length.

■ 5.2 CALCULATING STRESSES DUE TO APPLIED TORQUES

Shear stresses generated in structures resulting from applied torques are directly related to the magnitude of torque applied. The equation relating shear stress to torque is

$$\tau = \frac{Tr}{J} \quad \text{STRESSES IN TORSION} \tag{5.1}$$

where τ = shear stress
T = applied torque at section
r = distance from axis of twist to the point where shear stress is to be calculated
J = section shape parameter known as the polar moment of inertia

From this equation, one can see that shear stress is directly proportional to the torque applied to the section. In addition, if the location in the section where one wants to calculate stress is at the axis of twist, then $r = 0$, and the shear stress is equal to zero. This concurs with the basic concept of the axis of twist being the axis of zero stress in torsion.

> ➤ The *polar moment of inertia (J)* is a quantifiable parameter that describes the spatial distribution of the material in a structure section about its axis of twist. A sectional property of the structure, *J* is not related to the type of material from which the structure is made.

The final parameter in the equation for calculating stresses in torsion is the polar moment of inertia, J. J is a quantifiable parameter that reveals why some shapes resist twisting deformation better than others. It is related to the spatial distribution of material away from the axis of twist: The farther away the material from the axis of twist, the greater the structure's resistance to twisting. The concept of polar moment of inertia in determining torsional rigidity of a structure is very similar to the concept of area moment of inertia in determining bending rigidity. The units of J are length to the fourth power.

■ 5.3 DETERMINING POLAR MOMENT OF INERTIA (J)

Figure 5.3 lists the formulas for polar moments of inertia for several common shapes. Exact formulas are possible only for circular cross-

Shape	Polar Moment of Inertia, J
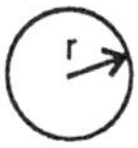 ⊙	$\dfrac{\pi}{2} r^4$
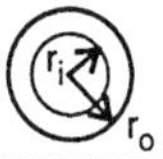 ⊚	$\dfrac{\pi}{2}(r_o^4 - r_i^4)$
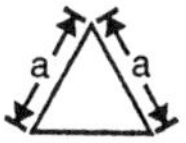 △	$\dfrac{\sqrt{3}}{80} a^4$
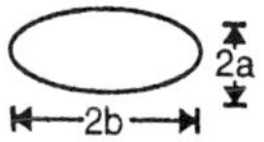 ⬭	$\dfrac{\pi\, a^3\, b^3}{a^2 + b^2}$
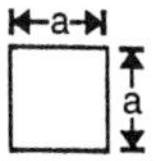 ▢	$0.1406\, a^4$

Figure 5.3. Formulas to calculate the polar moment of inertia for several common cross-section shapes. The formulas for nonaxisymmetric shapes are approximations only.

sections, but accurate approximations are available for noncircular shapes such as rectangles and triangles.

A structure's resistance to twisting deformation is referred to as its torsional rigidity. The more rigid a structure, the less it twists under a given torque. Just as in bending rigidity, torsional rigidity depends on the polar moment of inertia of the structure and the material stiffness in shear. Torsional rigidity of a structure made from a given material is defined by the factor GJ.

■ 5.4 DETERMINING STRESSES IN REAL STRUCTURES

As stated in equation 5.1, shear stresses in structures undergoing torsion are a function of the applied torque and structural geometry. To restate, the equation for determining stresses in torsion for structures composed of one material is

$$\tau = \frac{Tr}{J} \quad \text{SHEAR STRESS IN TORSION} \tag{5.1}$$

Just as in bending, stresses in torsion depend only on the applied torque and the size and shape of the structure, *not on the material from which the structure is manufactured*. An example of the use of this equation in orthopaedics is as follows:

Example: Fracture of a Skier's Tibia

Fracture of a skier's tibia can be caused by catching of the tip of the ski, thus creating a torque. If the skier's bindings are improperly set, they will not release appropriately, and the torque will be transmitted to the tibia at the top of the ski boot. When this happens, the tibia can break in a typical spiral fracture pattern. How much force would it take at the end of the ski to create such a fracture in a bone, as illustrated in figure 5.4? Assume a pure torque is applied to the tibia from the force on the ski, the cross-sectional geometry of the tibia is a hollow cylinder with dimensions as shown in figure 5.4, and the tibia fractures at a shear stress of 15,000 psi.

Solution. The maximum shear stress in the tibia is equal to Tr_o/J, as stated in equation 5.1. In this example,

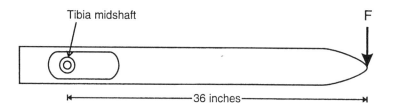

Tibia midshaft

F

←——————————— 36 inches ——————————→

r_o tibia = 0.52 inches
r_i tibia = 0.27 inches

Figure 5.4. A top view of a ski with boot mounted on it. The force applied at the end of the ski creates a large torque on the tibia because of the long moment arm created by the length of the ski.

$$T = F \times \text{moment arm} = F \times (36 \text{ inches})$$

$$r_o = 0.52 \text{ inches}, r_i = 0.27 \text{ inches}$$

$$J = \frac{\pi}{2}(r_o^4 - r_i^4) = (3.14/2)[(0.52 \text{ in})^4 - (0.27 \text{ in})^4]$$
$$= 0.1065 \text{ in}^4$$

$$\sigma_{\text{fracture}} = \frac{T_{\text{fracture}} r_o}{J} = \frac{T_{\text{fracture}}(0.52 \text{ in})}{(0.1065 \text{ in}^4)} = 15,000 \text{ psi}$$

$$T_{\text{fracture}} = \frac{15,000 \text{ psi} \times 0.1065 \text{ in}^4}{0.52 \text{ in}} = 3,072 \text{ in lb}$$

$$F_{\text{fracture}} = \frac{T_{\text{fracture}}}{36 \text{ inches}} = 85.4 \text{ lb}$$

From this calculation, one might assume that a force of 85.4 lb applied at the tip of the ski could generate sufficient torque to fracture the human tibia. Is this answer reasonable? Studies have shown that loads in this range applied to the end of a tightly bound ski can indeed cause fracture of the tibia. The fracture does not occur transversely but follows a spiral path. Why should this be so?

■ 5.5 SPIRAL FRACTURES IN TORSION

Take a piece of chalk and carefully twist it in pure torsion. The chalk will always fracture in a spiral fashion along a line about 45° from vertical, just like the tibial fracture in the previous example. Why does the chalk fracture at the 45° angle instead of making a nice transverse shear fracture with two flat surfaces? After all, shear is the primary stress associated with torsion. The reason has to do with how structures fail and the ease with which cracks that cause the failure can open and propagate.

In isotropic materials, cracks can open and propagate much more easily when pulled in tension than in shear. Figure 5.5a and b are illustrations of cracks opening in tension and shear, respectively. Imitate the opening of cracks in these two modes using your own fingers. It is much easier to spread two fingers apart than to slide them past each other. The same basic principle applies to cracks in materials. Because it is easier for cracks to open and propagate under tensile forces, it

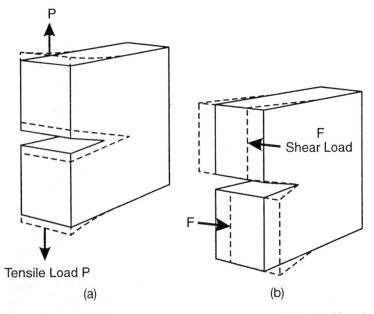

Figure 5.5. Cracks can open and extend due to tensile loads *(a)* and shear loads *(b)*. It is much easier to open a crack in tension.

makes sense that failure of structures almost always occurs from tensile stresses. (In chapter 16 we will discuss a few cases for which this may not be true.)

Thus the question remains: Why do spiral fractures occur in structures loaded in torque? To understand why this mode of failure occurs, one must look at the basic free-body diagram of the cylinder with applied torques as shown in figure 5.2. If another smaller, free-body diagram is made of just the small cube, as shown in figure 5.6, one can see that shear forces must act on each side face to keep the cube from rotating freely in space. The shear stress is equal to the magnitude of shear force divided by the area over which it acts.

Now split the cube in half along the diagonal and make another free-body diagram as shown in figure 5.7. If one resolves the forces along the surfaces of the body to satisfy static equilibrium and then calculates the stress on each face, one finds that the magnitude of the tensile stress on the diagonal face is equal to the magnitude of the shear stress! Because the tensile stress is more effective in opening and propagating defects, it will create failure along the 45° plane. (A detailed explanation of the resolution of forces is given as a note at the end of this chapter.)

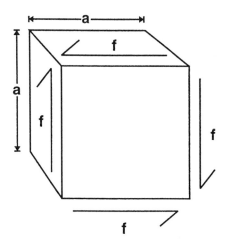

Figure 5.6. Shear forces must exist on all faces of a cube or it would rotate freely in space.

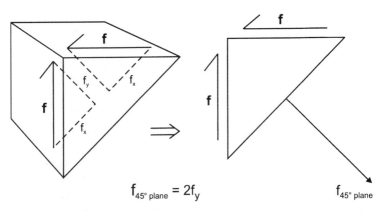

$$f_{45° \text{ plane}} = 2f_y$$

$$f_{45° \text{ plane}}$$

Figure 5.7. The tensile force at the 45° angle is equal to two times the *y* component of the shear force. If this force is divided by the area of the diagonal surface to determine stress, one finds that the tensile stress at the 45° plane is equal to the shear stress across the face of the cube.

The typical fracture progression of structures loaded in torsion is illustrated in figure 5.8a–d. Failure is initiated at a defect by the maximum tensile stress acting at 45° to the vertical (figure 5.8a). The crack continues to open from tension (figure 5.8b) until the crack wraps around to the opposite side (figure 5.8c). As the crack extends, the net section of remaining material becomes smaller and is off the axis of the applied torque. Complete fracture of the material occurs from bending of the net remaining section (figure 5.8d).

By knowing the mechanism by which fractures are created, one can often determine the loads, moments, and torques that will cause a structure's failure. For example, apply a clockwise pure torque to break a piece of chalk and compare the broken parts to a piece of chalk that was broken with a counterclockwise torque. The angle of fracture of the chalk broken with a counterclockwise torque is perpendicular to the fracture of the clockwise torque-fractured chalk (one is +45°; the other is −45°). Similarly, one can often determine the mechanism of injury of bone fractures by observing the fracture pattern. We discuss this subject further in chapter 9.

DETAILED EXPLANATION OF FORCE RESOLUTION OF THE 45° PLANE OF THE CUBE.   In figure 5.7, if one resolves each force, *f*, into its components (f_x along the diagonal surface and f_y perpendicular to this sur-

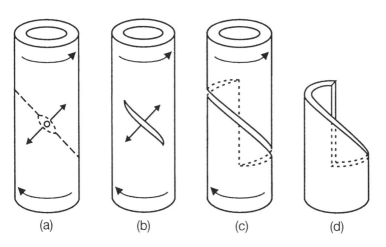

(a)   (b)   (c)   (d)

Figure 5.8. Steps of fracture progression of structures loaded in torsion. Failure initiates in maximum tension at 45° *(a)*, continues to open in tension *(b)* until the crack reaches the opposite side *(c)*. Finally the net remaining section is broken in off-axis bending *(d)*.

face), one will notice that the f_x components are in opposite directions and cancel each other, whereas the f_y components are in the same direction and add to give a resultant, $2f_y$, perpendicular to the diagonal surface. The stress that results from this force is a tensile stress acting across the diagonal surface and is equal to $2f_y$ divided by the area of the diagonal surface.

$$\sigma_{45° \text{ plane}} = \frac{2f_y}{A_{\text{diagonal}}}$$

but $f_x = f \times \sin 45°$ and $A_{\text{diagonal}} = 2A_{\text{side}} \times \cos 45°$.
Substituting:

$$\sigma_{45° \text{ plane}} = \frac{2f \sin 45°}{2A_{\text{side}} \cos 45°}$$

or

$$\sigma_{45° \text{ plane}} = \frac{f}{A_{\text{side}}} = \tau_{\text{side}}$$

Thus the tensile stress acting across the diagonal is equal in magnitude to the shear stress acting on the sides of the cube. Because defects tend to open into cracks under the influence of tensile stresses, these tensile stresses acting at 45° to the twist axis are responsible for the 45° spiral fractures characteristic of torsion failures.

Q5: Clinical Question (Summary)

Sandra Snowflake went skiing, took a tumble, and broke her leg. The break was a spiral fracture. Why does torsion create a tibial fracture?

A5: Clinical Answer

This question is answered in Section 5.5. When torsion is applied to a body, the shear stress on the 0° plane is equal to the tensile stress on the 45° plane. Because cracks are easier to open and propagate in tension, the tensile stresses will cause failure of the bone, and the crack (or fracture) will occur in the direction of maximum tension (i.e., along the 45° plane).

Additional Reading

Beer FP, Johnston ER: *Mechanics of Materials.* McGraw-Hill, New York, 1981.

Burstein AH, Wright TM: *Fundamentals of Orthopaedic Biomechanics.* Williams & Wilkins, Baltimore, 1994.

Orthopaedic Science: A Resource and Self-Study Guide for the Practitioner. American Academy of Orthopaedic Surgeons, Park Ridge, Ill., 1986 (ISBN 0-89203-011-9).

6

Stress Shielding of Bone

CLINICAL SCENARIO: BONE RESORPTION UNDER BONE PLATES

Instead of doing something dramatic (such as skiing) to break a bone, Fred Ferd tripped over the curb on the way to his car after work and fractured the midshaft of his radius and ulna. His fractures were treated the following day by open reduction and plating of both bones in the Swiss manner. His convalescence was uneventful, and his fractures healed in about 10 weeks, but subsequent X rays showed some resorption of the bone under the plates, and his surgeon began to suggest that the bone might not be as strong as he had hoped. What could cause bone under a rigid plate to suddenly begin to be absorbed?

Unlike other structural materials such as steel and plastic, bone is alive. When an engineer designs a bridge out of steel I beams, she does not have to worry about the ground at the base of the bridge resorbing if only a few people drive their cars across it. Such considerations do have to be made, however, in designing orthopaedic devices. Stress shielding of bone can be a major consideration in the design of implants and fracture fixation devices. In this chapter, we explore these concepts from the standpoint of the structural rigidity of an implant and its effect on tissues.

■ 6.1 ADAPTIVE REMODELING OF BONE: WOLFF'S LAW

It is common knowledge that bone and other tissues remodel according to the loads applied. The old saying "If you don't use it, you lose it!" has been applied to everything from the brain to muscles to other delicate neurological functions. In the late1800s, a German scientist named Julius Wolff published his now famous law, which stated that "every change in the form and function of bones or of their function alone is followed by certain definite changes in their configuration in accordance with mathematical laws." Today, *Wolff's law* is the term used generically to describe the response of bone to mechanical loads.

➢ Modernized Wolff's law: If you don't use it, you lose it with bone!

When a bone is subjected to stresses and strains substantially above or below its normal level, it responds by remodeling according to the new stresses applied. When a bone is shielded from stress, the bone mass will decrease; when subjected to higher than normal stresses (up to a point), the bone will respond by adding more material. The biological mechanisms that produce these effects are still poorly understood but reportedly involve electrical, chemical, and hormonal phenomena as well as mechanical processes at both the cellular and organ level.

Similarly, the concept of continuous mechanical repair of fatigue fractures of bone can help explain the phenomenon of Wolff's law. Bone is continuously repairing little cracks that occur naturally through repeated loading or fatigue. In normal loading of bone, these little cracks are repaired before they can cause a large-scale fracture. When bone is loaded at a strain level higher than normal, the rate of crack formation is higher, thus necessitating faster repair of the cracks (callus formation, or densification, of the bone) to avoid catastrophic failure. When the rate of crack formation exceeds the ability of the bone to repair itself, "stress fractures" occur. This type of injury is common in long-distance runners and military personnel who march for extended periods of time on hard surfaces.

■ 6.2 STRESS SHIELDING OF BONES BY IMPLANTS

When a fixation device or prosthesis is firmly attached to a bony structure, it will carry a portion of the load (perhaps a large portion) that would normally be carried by the intact skeleton if there were no abnormality requiring the implant. This stress sharing clearly means that the loads (and hence stresses and strains) in the adjacent bone will be reduced. If this stress reduction is great enough, it can induce atrophic remodeling (according to Wolff's law) that can lead to a loss of the prosthetic attachment or refracture of the bone adjacent to the fixation device. This type of reaction is often referred to as stress-shielding osteoporosis or stress-shielding osteopenia. Let us examine two examples of this phenomenon (a bone plate on a long bone and the proximal femur in total hip arthroplasty) from a strictly mechanical point of view, using the concepts presented in chapters 3, 4, and 5.

6.2.1 Bone Plates on a Long Bone

The idea of the implant, or device "carrying the load" away from the bone, is not foreign. In fact, one of the requirements of fracture-fixation devices is to reduce motion (and therefore load) at the fracture site so that the fracture can heal. What may be surprising to many, however, is the extent of load that a relatively small bone plate takes away from the bone.

The primary mode of loading in long bones is bending. As defined in chapter 4, in bending, the amount of strain (and therefore stress) depends on the bending rigidity of the section, EI. In a section composed of one material, this equation worked very well, but when a bone plate is added to a bone, the new section is composed of two materials with two different stiffnesses. The equations that deal with determining bending rigidity of a section composed of two materials can be complicated and are not required to understand the principles of the strain-shielding phenomenon; in this text, therefore, we approach the problem graphically.

First, consider the bone to be a hollow cylinder (figure 6.1a) and assume that a bending moment, M, is acting on it (figure 6.2a). In bending, the bone will assume a maximum stress, σ_{max} as follows:

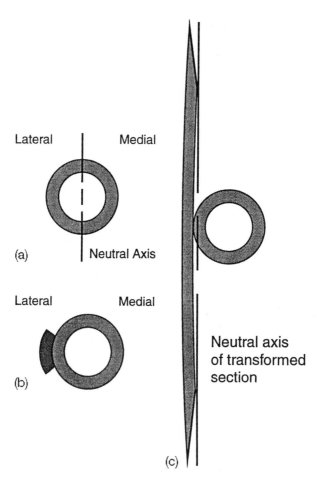

Figure 6.1. *(a)* A simplified cross section of a normal midshaft of a bone. If only bending moments are considered, the maximum tensile stress is at the lateral outer edge, maximum compression on the medial inner edge, and zero stress at the neutral axis. *(b)* Cross section of a bone with a bone plate (darker shading on lateral side); the neutral axis is no longer in the same place as in the original bone. *(c)* If the method of section transformation to equivalent materials is used, it is now obvious that the neutral axis shifts toward the lateral side, and the area moment of inertia of the bone with bone plate is much higher than that of the original bone.

$$\sigma_{max} = Mr_o/I_{bone}$$
$$= Mr_o/[(\pi/4)(r_o^4 - r_i^4)]$$

The maximum tensile strain in the bone, ε_{max}, is then

$$\varepsilon_{max} = \sigma_{max}/E_{bone}$$
$$= Mr_o/(E_{bone}I_{bone}).$$

When a bone plate is added (figures 6.1b and 6.2b), the calculation of the area moment of inertia of the combined section and of stress and strain is no longer so simple. However, a simple way of envisioning the effect of the bone plate on bending stresses is to imagine that the metal plate is replaced by a plate made of bone or at least some material with the same elastic modulus as bone. The new plate will then have an elastic modulus that is one-tenth that of the metal plate. If the new plate is to have the same rigidity as the metal plate, it will have to be 10 times as wide as the original metal plate (figure 6.1c). The advantage of making this imaginary change is that the entire structure in figure 6.1c is composed of the same material, so the rigidity factor, $EI,$ can now be applied to the system as a whole. If this is done, obviously the bone-and-plate combination has a much greater rigidity than the bone alone; thus, the strains in the bone with the plate will be much smaller. In fact, the lateral side of the original bone will now experience nearly zero stress under the bone plate because it is close to the neutral axis. The medial side of the bone will still experience compressive stresses on the order of previous stresses because of its increased distance from the neutral axis.

Figure 6.2 represents the A-P view of the bone with and without a bone plate under bending moment, M. From Wolff's law, one might predict that the bone remodeling that takes place would be bone resorption under the plate on the lateral side of the bone and slight changes (if any) on the medial side. At the ends of the plate, a section change occurs. As you will learn in chapter 8, a change in section causes a local increase in stress. Callus formation will occur in the bone at the ends of the plate. Figure 6.3 is a typical X ray of a bone that has had a bone plate applied for some period of time. Does the bone density distribution shown in the X ray correlate with our predictions?

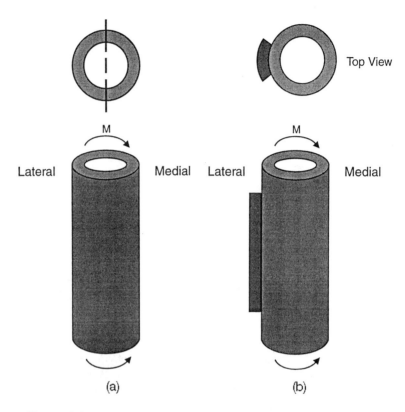

Figure 6.2. A bone midshaft under pure bending *(a)* and the same bone with a metal bone plate attached *(b)*.

6.2.2 Proximal Femur in Total Hip Arthroplasty

Placement of the metal femoral component in total hip arthroplasty can also lead to stress shielding of bone. Let us examine this situation in the same manner as with the bone plate.

Figure 6.4a shows a simplified cross section of the proximal femur in the region of the calcar. Assume that bending in the femur is the primary mode of loading and causes the neutral axis of the symmetric section to split the lateral and medial sides. When a femoral component is implanted, the new composite section can be shown (figure 6.4b). Notice that the neutral axis is not shifted in this case because the implant is assumed to be symmetric about the previous neutral axis.

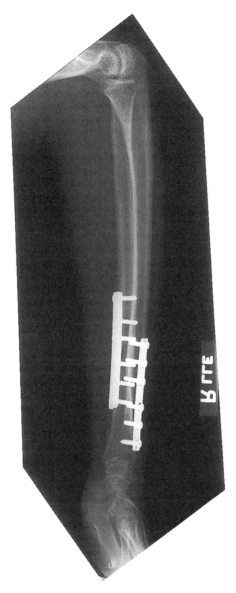

Figure 6.3. Early stress shielding under a forearm plate. Note also the adaptive change of the bone at the end of the plate where new bone is forming at some distance from the fracture site.

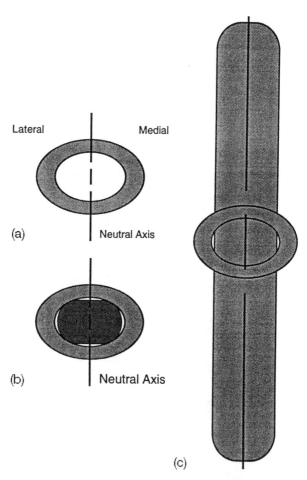

Figure 6.4. *(a)* A cross section of the calcar region of a proximal femur with the cancellous bone, which is of very low stiffness (not shown in order to simplify the problem). Assuming that the femur is subjected to pure bending, the neutral axis is in the middle of the section. *(b)* When a symmetric femoral prosthesis is implanted as shown, the neutral axis remains in the middle of the new section. *(c)* However, the area moment of inertia of the section is greatly increased by the large, stiff metal component. Therefore, stress across the entire section is greatly reduced as compared to normal.

By applying the same transformation-of-material idea that was used with the bone-plate situation, we can spread the cobalt-chromium-alloy implant along the neutral axis to make it 10 times longer but now made out of bone [$(E_{CoCr\text{-}alloy}/E_{bone}) = (200\ GPa/20\ GPa) = 10$] (figure 6.4c). Examine the section shown in figure 6.4c. The stress in the original bone (particularly at the calcar region) of the proximal femur will obviously be greatly lowered when an implant is inserted because the area

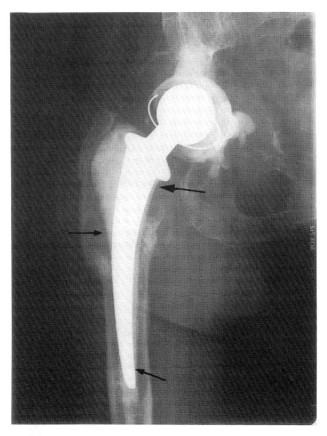

Figure 6.5. Severe loosening in a total hip arthroplasty that has given 15 years of service. Loosening is due to stress shielding (large arrow) at the calcar femorale and, more significantly, to particle-induced osteolysis (small arrows). What other patterns of remodeling are demonstrated in this radiograph?

moment of inertia of the transformed section is huge in comparison to the original bone. This stress shielding of the bone leads to a local reduction in bone mass as shown in the radiograph of figure 6.5. The total hip replacement in this radiograph has been in place for several years. The bone loss in this hip may be due to a combination of stress shielding and osteolysis from submicron polyethylene wear debris (see chapter 16).

Q6: CLINICAL QUESTION (SUMMARY)

Fred Ferd tripped on the curb and fractured the midshaft of his radius and ulna. His bones were plated in the Swiss manner but showed some resorption 10 weeks later. What could cause bone under a rigid plate to suddenly begin to adsorb?

A6: CLINICAL ANSWER

As discussed in Section 6.2.1 of this chapter, plating of a bone with a stiff plate can shield the bone from stress. According to the modernized Wolff's law, the bone was not used, so it lost some of its mass. Bone that is subjected to reduced stress or strain levels can be adsorbed within a relatively short period of time. Reduction of mass weakens the bone; Fred should definitely not try to curl a 50-pound dumbbell right after his plate is removed!

References

Bone Mechanics, SC Cowin, Ed., CRC Press, Boca Raton, Fla.,1989.

Huiskes R: Stress shielding and bone resorption in THA: Clinical versus computer-simulation studies. *Acta Orthop Belg* 59(S1):118–129, 1993.

Jacobs JJ, Sumner DR, Galante JO: Mechanisms of bone loss associated with total hip replacement. *Orthop Clin North Am* 24(4):583–590, 1993.

Martin RB, Burr DB: *Structure, Function and Adaptation of Compact Bone.* Raven Press, New York, 1989.

Roesler H: The history of some fundamental concepts in bone biomechanics. *J Biomech* 20(11/12):1025–1034, 1987.

Sumner DR, Galante JO: Determinants of stress shielding: Design versus materials versus interface. *Clin Orthop* 274:202–212, 1992.

Uhthoff HK, Foux A, Yeadon A, McAuley J, Black RC: Two processes of bone remodeling in plated intact femora: An experimental study in dogs. *J Orthop Res* 11(1):78–91, 1993.

7

Work and
Energy Concepts

CLINICAL SCENARIO: ENERGY IN JUMPING

Twenty-four-year-old Jack Jones, a second-year orthopaedic resident, had been a track star in the decalthalon when he went to undergraduate school at Wichita State University. During medical school at the University of Kansas, he concentrated on the high jump, practiced nearly every day, and even competed in the 1996 Olympic Games tryouts. He trained constantly, running sprints and jumping when the pit was available. But on becoming a resident with a more rigid and demanding schedule, he found it almost impossible to get in his daily workout and had to be content with a more erratic calendar of practicing. Sometimes he got up at 5 A.M. to work out and jump before early morning rounds at the hospital, or he worked out late at night after coming home from the hospital. Nevertheless, he did manage to train three or four times a week and thus burn up enough calories to allow him to cope with the hospital's food and maintain a weight of 65 kg. In his high jump, he did work and consumed energy. How much potential energy could he convert to kinetic energy by just barely clearing the six-and-a-half-foot high bar?

As used in the vernacular, the concepts of work and energy are often inconsistent with their strict mechanical definitions. "She spent a lot of mental energy in figuring out that problem" does not mean that she made her brain tissue consume a large amount of oxygen! Similarly, comparing the concepts of mechanical and biological energy expenditures and work can be confusing. In this chapter, we examine the basic ideas of work and energy from both the mechanical and biological points of view.

■ 7.1 DEFINITION OF WORK AND ENERGY

By definition, *work* is the product of a force times the distance through which the force acts. This implies that the force and distance must be in the same direction. For example, to lift a box of books weighing 100 N a total of 1 m off of the floor, as in figure 7.1, the total work done by the mover is 100 N m. Similarly, when a person walks up a flight of stairs, the work done is equal to the ground reaction force times the vertical distance traveled. No work is associated with an automobile's forward motion, however, because the ground reaction force (force of gravity) is perpendicular to the motion direction. In muscles, the direction of movement of the muscle during its contractile phase is coincident with the direction of the muscle force. Therefore, the muscle performs work on the body during contraction.

Work = Force × Distance

In the SI system, the units of work are newtons times meters, or joules. One joule equals 1 N m, or, in other words, 1 J equals the work performed by a force of 1 N moving through a distance of 1 m.

➢ *Work* is the product of force times the distance through which the force acts.

➢ *Energy* is the ability to do work.

Energy can be defined as the ability to perform work and has the same units as work. Energy has many different forms. In figure 7.1, the

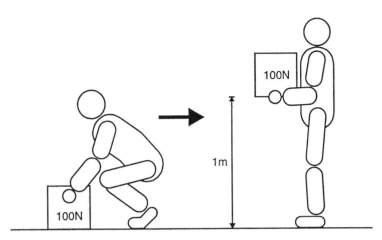

Figure 7.1. A mover lifts a box of books weighing 100 N 1 m off the floor. The total work done by the mover is the force times the vertical distance, which equals 100 N m.

mover did work in lifting the box and placing it on a table 1 m above the ground. This work is now stored in the elevated box in the form of potential energy, and this energy can be recovered in an equivalent amount of work done if the box is lowered to the ground. In its most common form, *potential energy* is the energy stored when a weight is raised against the force of gravity above a stable surface. Potential energy is equal to the product of the weight of the box and its distance above the stable surface (in this case, the floor).

Potential Energy = Weight × Height

If the box is dropped to the floor, it no longer possesses potential energy because it has given up its elevation. However, energy is always conserved; the potential energy of the box is not lost but converted to a different form. Just before hitting the floor, the box has a finite velocity and therefore possesses *kinetic energy,* or the energy of movement. Kinetic energy is by definition the product of one-half the mass of the object and the square of the velocity at which it is traveling.

Kinetic Energy $= \frac{1}{2} \times$ Mass $\times$ Velocity^2

As the box is falling, the height of the box is decreasing (therefore, potential energy is decreasing), and the velocity is increasing (therefore, kinetic energy is increasing). When the box hits the floor, energy is transferred by pushing against the floor and doing work on it. By pushing down on the floor, the box is deforming the floor (however slightly). It is hoped that, for the person standing next to the box, the floor experiences only elastic deformation and has the ability to spring back to its original shape. The kinetic energy was then transformed into *strain energy,* or the energy associated with deformation.

➤ Strain energy is the energy of deformation.

The type of floor affects the response of the box as it hits the surface. A very hard floor surface will transmit nearly all the strain energy back to the box and do work on it; the box may even bounce in response to the work being done on it. A soft surface will absorb some or all of the strain energy and will, in effect, "soften the blow" of the box hitting the surface because not as much work will be returned to the box by the surface. Ultimately, all the energy converted into elastic deformation of the floor and the box itself is converted into heat and sound (noise), which are dissipated into the surroundings.

7.1.1 Energy of Falls

People who are standing also have potential energy by virtue of the fact that their center of gravity is maintained at a distance above the floor's surface. If a person falls, the impact that he or she experiences (or the energy the body has to absorb) depends on the distance from the surface, body weight, and the energy-absorbing capability of the surface. The old saying, "the bigger they are, the harder they fall," really does hold true!

At first glance, one might translate these concepts into "heavier people are more likely to break their hips when they fall." In fact, that may not be the case. With regard to fractures, one must consider the entire energy-absorption capability of the body. When a thin woman falls, the bone of the proximal femur is not protected by much energy-absorbing material. Yes, the energy of impact is less, but the energy generated is transmitted mainly to the bone. Fat is a good energy-absorbing material. When a heavier woman falls, the energy of the impact is greater, but the fat around her hip can absorb some of the energy of the impact; the result is that less is transferred to the bone of the proximal femur. In addition, the heavier woman may have Wolff's law in her favor with more dense bone from higher everyday loading. Indeed, it is possible that the thin woman is more likely to break her hip than the heavier woman from a fall at the same height.

7.1.2 Energy of Impact Injuries

A high kinetic energy is associated with a high-velocity-impact injury. Because energy is conserved, the kinetic energy is transferred to the soft and hard tissues, resulting in great soft tissue disruption and a high degree of comminution of the bone. This subject is discussed in detail in chapter 9.

■ 7.2 WORK AND ENERGY CONCEPTS IN GAIT

As human animals, we exist through the conversion of chemical energy into mechanical energy. We eat food as a source of energy that is either used immediately or stored as "love handles." The stored chemical energy of food is metabolized as a sort of gas for our body engine. Our metabolism of this energy, or conversion of the energy of food, starts with the oxidation of nutrients. The energy expended, or energy cost during a specific activity, can therefore be determined indirectly by measuring oxygen consumption during that activity. The rate of oxygen consumption is the most common means of describing energy costs. For ambulation, oxygen consumption is reported as either the net oxygen cost in milliliters of O_2 per kilogram-meter to show the energy cost related to mobility, or by the rate of oxygen uptake in milliliters of O_2 per kilogram-minute as the cost of maintaining a specific performance level for a given period of time. Net oxygen cost is considered to be the best way to compare the efficiencies of different types of gait.

The most common way to describe energy consumption in the general population is by calorie consumption. A calorie (or gram-calorie) is the basic unit of heat energy and is defined as the amount of heat necessary to raise the temperature of 1 g of water 1°C. Physical energy expenditure can be measured by direct calorimetry or by determining the body's heat and work production. However, this type of measurement is complex and impractical for most laboratory experiments. Measurement of the oxygen consumption provides an indirect determination of energy expenditure that is simpler and more practical.

7.2.1 Gait Efficiency

Every time we take a step in level walking, we move our center of gravity up and down through a cyclic pattern (figure 7.2). The vertical oscillation of the center of gravity corresponds to changes in the potential energy of the body. The potential energy is high when the center of gravity is high and low when the center of gravity is low. An increment of work is done every time the center of gravity goes from low to high. Metabolic energy is required to bring the center of gravity up to its original position, but this energy is not utilized in moving the body forward. Efficient gait therefore involves minimization of the vertical excursion of the center of gravity of the body between steps.

We can clarify the concepts of changing center of gravity by contrasting the energy expended when walking uphill and downhill. When one walks downhill, the natural eventual lowering of the body's center of gravity creates a greater-than-normal amount of potential energy, which can be converted into kinetic energy. In contrast, walking uphill increases the potential energy required to maintain the usual height of the center of gravity. Therefore, walking uphill requires an increase in metabolic energy (that is, some huffing and puffing) to increase oxygen uptake. The shifting center-of-gravity concept is illustrated in figure 7.3.

The energy expenditure due to the vertical motion is only a part of the overall energy required to walk. Energy is required for many other activities, such as acceleration and deceleration of the legs in swinging, impact of the foot with the ground, and other dynamic effects. The *efficiency* of the gait process can be defined as the percentage of energy input that is transformed into useful work. Studies have shown that humans can achieve an efficiency of only about 20%–30%. Because we

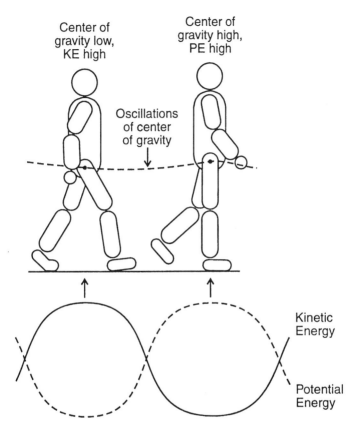

Figure 7.2. Every time we walk, we move our center of gravity (CG) in vertical oscillations. When the CG is at a low point, the kinetic energy is high; when the CG is at a high point, the potential energy is high. *Source:* Cochran GVB: *A Primer of Orthopaedic Biomechanics.* Churchill Livingstone, New York, 1982, p. 282.

are subject to the law of conservation of energy, the portion of the energy that is not employed in locomotion is converted to heat.

7.2.2 Efficiency of Abnormal Gait

Our internal engine then uses metabolically produced "gasoline" to propel us. But what if a person's tire gets a flat? Abnormalities in an in-

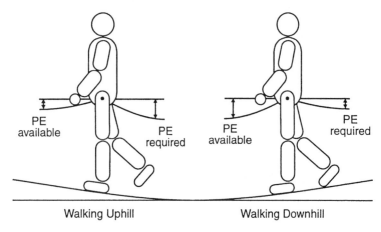

Walking Uphill   Walking Downhill

Figure 7.3. When one walks up a hill, more potential energy is required than is available; thus energy must be input from the body. Conversely, when one goes downhill, the available potential energy is greater than the required amount. *Source:* Cochran GVB: *A Primer of Orthopaedic Biomechanics.* Churchill Livingstone, New York, 1982, p. 282.

dividual's extremities will disturb the gait cycle and increase the gait-energy expenditure. For example, studies have shown that average energy expenditure increases by 10% when a short leg brace is worn, by 25% when a person has a stiff knee, and by up to 60% when walking speed is increased.

In amputees, studies have shown that test subjects decrease their gait velocity to keep the rate of energy expenditure within normal limits. The slower walking speed is a measure of the loss of efficiency. The best way to compare an amputee's gait-energy expenditure to normal values is by comparing the net oxygen cost in milliliters of O_2 per kilogram-meter. On average, energy expenditure is increased by 60% with a below-knee amputation and by 100% by an above-knee amputation.

Similarly, the energy costs of ambulation are higher for patients with arthritis. One study found that the energy cost for patients with osteoarthritis prior to total knee replacement was 55% higher than for patients without arthritis. Patients with rheumatoid arthritis using no assist device had a 170% higher energy cost than normal prior to surgery. If the patient used a walker to assist in ambulation, his or her energy costs were 320% higher than normal. After unilateral total knee replacement, all patients exhibited a significantly lower energy cost of ambulation. After total knee replacement surgery, rheumatoid patients had energy costs only 25% higher than normal patients without arthritis. Total knee replacement surgery reduced the energy costs for rheumatoid patients who still required the assistance of a walker by over 55% compared to their presurgery condition.

Q7: CLINICAL QUESTION (SUMMARY)

Dr. Jack Jones was practicing his high jump on an erratic schedule. Three to four times a week he worked out and managed to maintain a weight of 65 kg despite the "free food on call" tickets for the hospital cafeteria. How much potential energy did he convert to kinetic energy by just barely clearing the six-and-a-half-foot high bar?

A7: CLINICAL ANSWER

Dr. Jones certainly beat the odds by being able to maintain his trim 65-kg weight while on call. The work he did to clear the bar in his high jump was equal to the force of gravity acting on his 65-kg body multiplied by the height of his jump of 6.5 ft. Converting kilograms to newtons (multiply by 9.8) and feet to meters (multiply by 0.3048), we have

$$\text{Work} = 65 \text{ kg } (9.8 \text{ N/kg}) \times 6.5 \text{ ft } (0.3048 \text{ m/ft})$$

$$\text{Work} = 1262 \text{ N m} = \text{Potential energy}$$

Additional Reading

Cochran GVB: *A Primer of Orthopaedic Biomechanics.* Churchill Livingstone, New York, 1982.

Perry J: *Gait analysis: Normal and Pathological Function.* SLACK, Thorofare, N.J., 1992.

Torburn L, Powers CM, Gutierrez R, Perry J: Energy expenditure during ambulation in dysvascular and traumatic below-knee amputees: A comparison of five prosthetic feet. *J Rehabil Res Dev* 32(2):111–119, 1995.

Waters RL, Campbell J, Thomas L, Hugos L, Davis P: Energy costs of walking in lower-extremity plaster casts. *J Bone Joint Surg* 64A(6):896–899, 1982.

Waters RL, Perry J, Conaty P, Lunsford B, O'Meara P: The energy cost of walking with arthritis of the hip and knee. *Clin Orthop* 214:278–284, 1987.

8

Stress Raisers, Fracture, and Fatigue

CLINICAL SCENARIO: TWO BONE PLATES CLOSE TOGETHER

Sixty-eight-year-old Martha Mainstream had a replacement arthroplasty for her hip three years ago for severe osteoarthritis. Because she no longer had to utilize a cane to get around, the op-

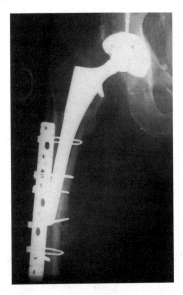

Figure 8.1. Radiograph of a large bone plate applied across a fracture below a prosthetic femoral stem.

eration changed her life, and she was relieved of the nearly constant pain in her groin and down her thigh. As a matter of fact, she had resumed walking and swimming for exercise and had lost 20 pounds of excess weight. Alas, when she went out to feed her cats, she slipped on some wet grass and sustained a fracture of her femur well below the prosthetic femoral stem. She underwent surgery again and had a large bone plate applied across the fracture, shown in figure 8.1. What problems are likely to arise from having two metal devices close together in this fashion?

Everything eventually fails; it is just a question of how, when, and why. In chapters 3, 4, and 5, you learned about stress from an engineering point of view. In this chapter, you will learn what causes fracture in materials and what prevents even materials and structures developed for military purposes from being all that they can be.

■ 8.1 STRESS-RAISING DEFECTS

Stress-raising defects are defined as holes, voids, cracks, and so on (usually on the microscopic level) that act locally to increase the stress on objects under tension. In order to understand the nature of stress raisers, we first examine them in the macroscopic sense as design aspects of structures.

Stress-concentration Factor, K

$$K = \sigma_{peak}/\sigma_{average}$$

Consider the bone plate shown schematically in figure 8.2a. Obviously, the stress near the hole (section A-A′) is larger than the stress in the through section (B-B′) just because the cross-sectional area is reduced by the hole. However, the stress near the hole is even greater than one would expect on considering just reduction of area. The stress distribution across the remaining section near the hole is not even but is

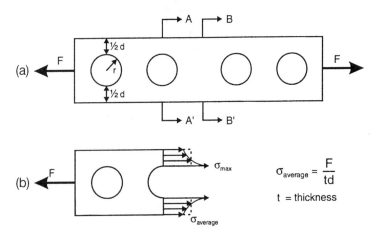

Figure 8.2. *(a)* A bone plate is in tension under normal conditions in the body. The stresses in the plate are greater at the location of the screw holes (A-A') than at the whole section (B-B'), not only because of the reduced cross section but also because of the stress-raising effect of the hole. The distribution of the increased stress is shown in *(b)*.

greatest at the edge of the hole and gradually decreases as the distance from the hole increases (figure 8.2b). The stress-raising effect of the hole can be characterized by a term called the stress-concentration factor (SCF). The stress-concentration factor, usually referred to by the letter *K,* is the ratio between the peak stress at the defect and the average stress over the section.

The magnitude of the SCF depends on the shape and size of the defect. For example, figure 8.3 gives the stress-concentration factors for different sizes of circular holes and fillets in a plate under tension. Notice that the SCF (or *K*) increases rapidly for sharp transitions. For the bone plate in figure 8.2, one might guess that the stress-concentration factor for the relatively large hole in the small plate would be around two because the ratio of the radius of the hole to the net section on one side *(r/d)* is about one. In other words, the maximum stress in the structure (due to the stress-concentrating effect of the hole) is about two times what one would have predicted from a simple stress analysis using the tensile-stress equation of load divided by area.

Now consider defects on a microscopic scale. In the manufacture of real materials, small defects such as trapped gas bubbles or contami-

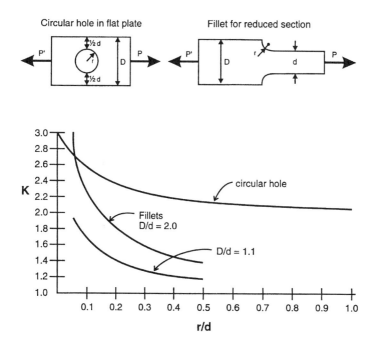

Figure 8.3. Typical stress-concentration factors for plates with holes and reduced sections with fillets are given as a function of the relative size of the parts. Notice that for the reduced section part, the sharper the fillet and the greater the section change, the higher the stress-concentration effect. *Source:* Beer FP, Johnston ER: *Mechanics of Materials.* McGraw-Hill, New York, 1981, p. 81, Figure 2.59.

nants are always created. For analysis of the effect of these types of defects, we find it helpful to consider the type of material containing the defect. In general, homogeneous isotropic materials can be separated into classifications of brittle and ductile in determining the effect of a stress raiser.

8.1.1 Stress-Raising Defects in Brittle Materials

Materials that exhibit little or no plastic deformation before they fracture are referred to as brittle materials. Some examples of this type of material are ceramics, glasses, and a few polymers like the polymethyl-methacrylate (PMMA) bone cement. Brittle materials are particularly sensitive to stress-raising defects. If brittle materials are made without defects, they may be extremely strong; however, this is very difficult (if not impossible) and very expensive to achieve. Theories have been developed to explain (and predict) the fracture stress of brittle materials. Perhaps the first person to recognize and help explain the nature of stress-raising defects was A. A. Griffith. In 1920 Griffith calculated the theoretical strength of glass according to the strength of the molecular bonds. He noticed that the ultimate tensile strength of bulk glass was much lower than the theoretical strength. Griffith went on to make smaller samples of glass down to very thin drawn-glass fibers. He found that after a certain point, as the diameter of the glass specimen decreased, the tensile strength increased until the drawn-glass fiber nearly reached the theoretical strength. Through further analysis, he found that the fibers were nearly void free, and he was able to show that flaws in the bulk glass were responsible for the reduction of strength.

> ➢ Brittle materials are very sensitive to stress-raising defects.

Unlike human beings, not all cracks are created equal. The size and shape of a crack determine its stress-raising effect. Griffith developed a theory to explain the effect of the size and shape of cracks in brittle materials. For a small elliptical defect in a large plate under tension (figure 8.4), Griffith found that the stress-concentration factor of the ellipse was a function of the ratio of the crack length and height such that $K = 1 + 2c/b$. For example, for the ellipse in figure 8.4, which has dimensions c/b of about 5/1, the stress at the edge of the ellipse would be about 11 times the average stress in the material. Clearly, a very sharp, long crack can create dangerously high stress concentrations in a structure. In fact, that is one reason why cracks in glass windshields propagate so rapidly and why scratching a strong glass rod makes it very easy to break. Consider the effect of a circular defect in a large plate. Does the stress-concentration factor predicted by Griffith's equation agree with the empirical data shown in figure 8.3?

The orientation of the defect with respect to the direction of tension is important. The elliptical hole of figure 8.4 turned 90° so that it runs

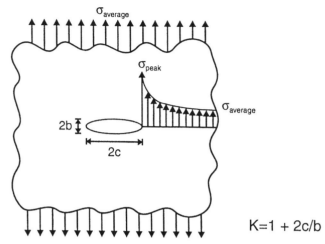

Figure 8.4. An elliptical defect in a large plate will experience a stress-concentration factor, *K*, that is governed by the shape of the defect according to the formula $K = 1 + 2c/b$ with a general stress distribution as shown. What would be the stress-concentration factor for a circular hole ($b = c$)? Does this agree with the data shown in figure 8.3?

along the direction of the applied tensile stress is not very severe at all, with a stress concentration now of 1.4 (about 1/10 the previous stress concentration). It is not just the shape and size of the defect that matters but also its orientation with respect to the tensile loading.

It should now be obvious why brittle materials are very strong in compression but not in tension. In compression, the small flaws are forced together, and there is no stress-concentration effect. Therefore, the compressive strength of a brittle material approaches the ideal. For tensile loading, a knowledge of the size range and rate of occurrence of preexisting flaws in brittle materials can be used to predict the range of average stresses over which fracture will occur. The modern quantitative analysis of brittle fracture in structural components is called *fracture mechanics*.

8.1.1.1 Reducing the Effect of a Defect in Brittle Materials

With the exception of PMMA bone cement, brittle materials (like ceramics) are not used to any great extent in orthopaedics even though they may be very strong and biocompatible. The risk of brittle fracture of such a device due to defects (inherent in the material or created during surgery) in high stress applications is a major concern. Techniques have been developed to reduce the risk of fracture in devices made from brittle materials. Fire polishing of the surface of the part smoothes and rounds any existing surface cracks. Another technique is the creation of residual compressive stresses in the surface that have to be overcome before tensile stresses are formed in the component. These techniques are currently used in making the ceramic ball for the femoral component of a total hip system. These devices are used clinically and are safe and work well; however, a ceramic femoral head can break if it is scratched when dropped on the floor (see chapter 13).

8.1.2 Stress-Raising Defects in "Forgiving" Materials

In contrast to brittle materials (such as ceramics) that are very sensitive to defects, some materials are less sensitive to stress-raising defects. Ductile materials (such as most metals and many plastics) also experience an initial high-stress concentration due to a sharp crack. However, these materials can deform to absorb energy away from the crack tip, blunt the crack, and therefore reduce the stress concentration (figure 8.5). Brittle materials are sensitive to stress-raising defects because

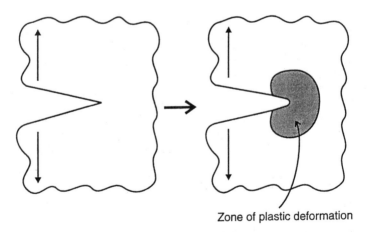

Zone of plastic deformation

Figure 8.5. The region of plastic deformation (and therefore energy absorption) in front of the crack is shaped somewhat like a lima bean. This plastic deformation will help draw energy away from the crack tip. In addition, the blunting of the crack tip during plastic deformation will reduce the stress-concentration effect of the crack.

they do not have the capability for plastic deformation and related energy absorption and cannot reduce the effect of the stress concentration.

➤ Ductile materials are not very sensitive to stress-raising defects.

One measure of the resistance of a material to fracture in the presence of a sharp defect is fracture toughness. The fracture toughness of a material is measured by inducing a very sharp crack in a standard-sized specimen and measuring the load required to break the material in comparison to the crack length. Materials with a high fracture-toughness value absorb a lot of energy before failing in the presence of a defect, whereas materials with lower fracture toughness do not and tend toward brittle behavior.

8.1.3 Defects in Bone

Graft removal, reconstruction, and other surgical procedures often create defects in bone. Although bone (discussed in chapter 17) is a complex material, it is useful to treat it initially as a homogeneous structural unit like an I beam in a bridge or a column in a building. Defects with high aspect ratios and sharp cracklike features oriented perpendicular to the direction of tensile stresses will yield high stress concentrations. Figure 8.6 shows the sites from which three types of bones grafts have been removed with square corner ends, rounded corner ends, and elliptical ends. Reducing the stress-raising effect of the defect by eliminating sharp corners and increasing the curvature makes the oval-shaped end more appropriate for graft removal.

8.1.4 Effect of Section Change and Proximity of Defects

In chapter 6, the concept of the rigidity of a structure made from multiple materials was introduced. In Section 6.2.1, we mentioned that callus formation occurs near the ends of a bone plate due to the local increase in stress. Whenever the cross section of a structure changes abruptly, a stress-concentration effect will result. The ends of a bone plate and the distal tip of a femoral-hip-prosthesis component are two

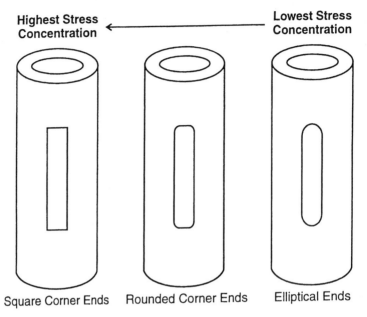

Highest Stress Concentration ← **Lowest Stress Concentration**

Square Corner Ends   Rounded Corner Ends   Elliptical Ends

Figure 8.6. A bone with three types of defects. Of these three defect shapes (square corner ends, rounded corner ends, and elliptical, or oval, ends) the elliptical ends yield the lowest stress-concentration effect.

classic examples of section changes in orthopaedics that lead to stress concentrations.

Neither the stress increase at the bone plate ends nor that at the tip of the femoral component is generally large enough to cause problems such as bone fracture. However, if two components are in proximity, the stress concentrations caused by each individual component can add together, possibly raising the local stress to dangerous levels. Examples of this undesirable situation would be the placing of two bone plates end-to-end or putting a bone plate near the distal tip of a femoral component. In such circumstances, the combined stress enhancements might eventually cause failure of the bone due to fatigue fracture (see Section 8.3).

Stress-concentration effects from defects in proximity can also add together to create higher stresses than anticipated from the individual defects. For example, two holes close together can actually act as one

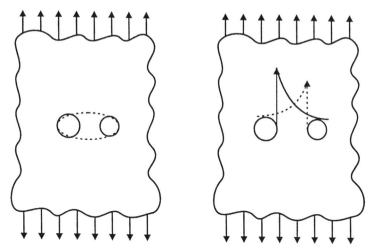

Figure 8.7. If two defects are in proximity, either they may appear to be one large defect and therefore have a greater stress-raising effect or the individual stress-raising effects of the two defects might add together.

much larger elliptical hole that produces a larger stress concentration than the individual circular holes (figure 8.7). This is a real concern in the bone-cement mantle of a joint replacement. Several small bubble defects can produce a large stress concentration that can initiate fracture.

■ 8.2 STATIC FRACTURE OF MATERIALS AND STRUCTURES

Static fracture (or, more correctly, quasi-static fracture) occurs when a structure under one-time loading suddenly breaks. An example of static fracture would be the fluke fracture of a ceramic ball of a femoral component that slipped out of a surgeon's hands and landed "just wrong" on the surgery-suite floor. Much can be learned from the fracture surface. With much training and experience, one can determine the relative quality of the material (for example, whether manufacturing flaws were present), the defect(s) that precipitated the fracture, and other important information. Fortunately, static fracture of orthopaedic devices is rarely the mode of failure. Only if there were severe manufacturing defects or grossly inappropriate use or misplacement of the device would fracture from one-time loading occur. For this reason, analysis of static fracture is not covered in this book. Many excellent references on this subject are available if you have further interest.

■ 8.3 FATIGUE FAILURE OF MATERIALS AND STRUCTURES

Nearly every mechanical failure of orthopaedic materials and devices is caused by gradual extension of a crack until complete fracture occurs. This process is called fatigue or fatigue failure. The fatigue process involves repeated loading to stress levels below the UTS; in fact, the stresses are often only a small fraction of the yield stress. At such low stress levels, nothing happens on the first loading cycle or for many cycles thereafter. With a sufficient number of cycles, however, a microcrack eventually forms. The number of cycles required to first form a crack is called the initiation period.

Once the crack is present, successive loading cycles cause it to advance or "jump ahead" in microsteps, one step per load cycle. The period of advancement is referred to as propagation. The steps, or fatigue striations, can be readily identified in the scanning electron microscope and can sometimes be seen without magnification. The steps of fatigue striations look like and are referred to as a clamshell pattern because they start out small and gradually get larger and extend in the shape of the plastic zone. When the crack has propagated through enough of the cross section so that the intact portion remaining can no longer carry the service loads, complete failure occurs. When the stem of the femoral component of a hip prosthesis fails, or when the plate or screws from a fixation system fail in association with a protracted nonunion, fatigue has usually been found responsible. However, sometimes rubbing of the fracture surfaces in vivo after failure obliterates the striations.

Much can be learned about why a part broke from the fatigue striations and fracture surface. A wonderful example of this is shown in figure 8.8. This photograph shows the handle and fracture surface of a hairbrush that a rather thick-haired first-year resident brought into our laboratory after finishing his biomechanics rotation. His brush broke one day with no prior warning, but, as you can see, the fatigue crack

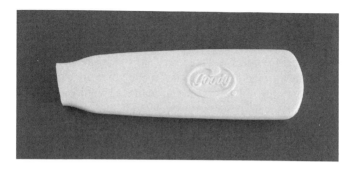

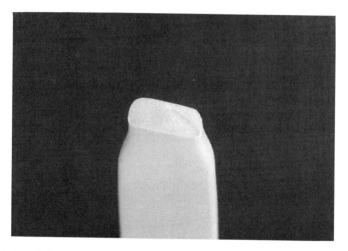

Figure 8.8. Photograph of the front of a brush handle (logo on bristle side) and top view of a thick-haired resident's brush that broke with no warning. Where and why did the fatigue fracture initiate?

had been developing for some time before final failure. By examination of the fracture surface and knowing that cracks open due to tension, can you tell whether the resident is right or left handed? (Hint: Try using an imaginary brush handle to brush your own hair, determine what side is in tension, and then observe how the fatigue striation [clamshell] pattern has developed. The brush logo is on the bristle side of the handle.)

All structural materials—metals, ceramics, polymers, and composites—are subject to fatigue. The fatigue of metals has received the most attention from materials scientists because metals are usually reserved for the most highly stressed and critical applications.

To study the fatigue behavior of metals (and other materials), a number of identical specimens are prepared. The specimens are divided into several groups, and all the specimens in one group are exposed to the same cyclical stress. The cycles are continued until each specimen breaks; then the average number of cycles to failure at that stress is calculated. The next group is exposed to a different stress level. This process is continued until the average cycles to failure has been determined for stresses from the yield stress to about 1/4 of the yield stress. Such plots are called S-N (stress versus number) curves. Figure 8.9 is a typical S-N curve for the titanium alloy Ti 6Al, 4V.

From figure 8.9, it is obvious that the number of cycles to failure increases rapidly as the maximum stress per cycle is reduced. Furthermore, when the stress is low enough, it often appears that failure will not occur even after an unlimited number of cycles. This stress is called the *endurance,* or *fatigue, limit.* For the hot forged and low temperature annealed bar in figure 8.9, it appears that the endurance limit is a little less than 700 MPa. It is standard engineering practice to design load-

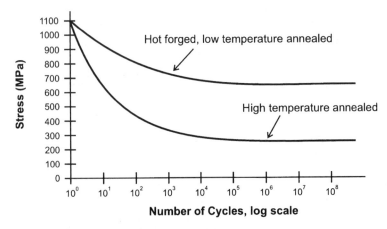

Figure 8.9. A stress versus number of cycles (S-N) curve is for a titanium alloy (metal) with two different types of heat treatment. In some cases such as this one, the type of heat treatment used in processing the part can dramatically change the fatigue response of the material.

bearing structures so that the average service stresses are below this endurance limit. This is usually accomplished by increasing the size of the part. In some cases, this may be difficult to do because there is a weight limitation (spacecraft) or a size limitation (diameter of the femoral medullary cavity).

➢ *Endurance limit,* or *fatigue limit,* is the stress level below which fatigue failure of the material will not occur.

In addition, many factors may reduce the endurance limit of an alloy. In figure 8.9, it is obvious that heat treatment during the manufacturing process can produce changes that reduce the endurance limit by about 250 MPa or by 35% for the high-temperature treated (annealed) material. This is important in the clinical use of the Ti 6Al-4V alloy with a porous coating. The treatment by which the beads are bonded to the surface (called sintering) is equivalent to the high-temperature anneal and produces comparable lowering of the endurance limit. Furthermore, the "necks" by which the beads are attached to the substrate involve sharp notches with stress-concentration-factor values up to 4. The combination of stress concentration and the reduced fatigue life of the material as a result of heat treatment can lead to catastrophic failure of the device if the problem is not addressed.

In order to understand the fatigue phenomenon, one must first realize that all crack extension leading to fracture is an energy-related process. A certain amount of strain energy must be put into the system for the crack to open and create new surfaces with their own surface energy. Whenever the energy required to extend the crack is reduced, the number of cycles to fail the material is reduced. In the case of the titanium alloy previously referred to, the high-temperature annealed (treated) material had a reduced fatigue resistance because the grains of its microstructure were large and flat, and the cracks propagated easily along the grain boundaries. (Chapter 14 discusses this general problem as well as metal microstructure.)

Fracture and fatigue mechanisms are complicated fields of study, and a great deal about these fields (such as the effect of complicated spectrum loading on crack propagation) is not yet completely understood. For this reason, mechanical testing of devices (including fatigue testing) is always required before they can be used clinically. The factors to be considered in mechanical testing of orthopaedic devices and materials are covered in chapter 12.

By the way, the thick-haired first-year resident was right handed.

Q8: CLINICAL QUESTION (SUMMARY)

Martha Mainstream, proud owner of a total hip, had a distal femoral fracture on the same leg fixed with a bone plate. What problems are likely to arise from having two implants close together in this fashion?

A8: CLINICAL ANSWER

As discussed in Section 8.1.4, a sudden change in the load-bearing cross section (such as at the end of a bone plate or tip of the hip implant) will cause an increase in stress. The effect is further increased when two such section changes occur in proximity. As a result, placing the end of the plate close to the tip of the prosthesis greatly increases the likelihood of overloading of the bone, leading to fatigue failure and fracture. Although this is not a guaranteed outcome for Martha's femur, the probability is relatively high. Overlapping of implants should thus be avoided.

Additional Reading

Beer FP, Johnston ER: *Mechanics of Materials.* McGraw-Hill, New York, 1981.

Davies JP, Burke DW, O'Connor DO, Harris WH: Comparison of the fatigue characteristics of centrifuged and uncentrifuged Simplex P bone cement. *J Orthop Res* 5:366–371, 1987.

Davies JP, Harris WH: Effect of hand mixing tobramycin on the fatigue strength of Simplex P. *J Biomed Mater Res* 25:1409–1414, 1991.

Hertzberg RW: *Deformation and Fracture Mechanics of Engineering Materials,* 3rd ed. John Wiley & Sons, New York, 1989.

James SP, Jasty M, Davies JP, Piehler H, Harris WH: A fractographic investigation of PMMA bone cement focusing on the relationship between porosity reduction and increased fatigue life. *J Biomed Mater Res* 26:651–662, 1992.

Sih GC, Berman AT: Fracture toughness concept applied to methyl methacrylate. *J Biomed Mater Res* 14:311–324, 1980.

Topoleski LDT, Ducheyne P, Cuckler JM: Microstructural pathway of fracture in poly(methyl methacrylate) bone cement. *Biomaterials* 14(15):1165–1172, 1993.

9

Biomechanics of Pathology

CLINICAL SCENARIO: STRENGTH OF A BONE WITH A TUMOR

Martha Mainstream's twin sister Matilda also had pain in her groin and in the thigh, but this had been a problem for only a couple of months. The discomfort was so persistent at night that she had great difficulty turning over in bed. Matilda had no cats to feed; she simply fell in her kitchen—or more accurately, her leg collapsed, causing her to fall. When she arrived at the hospital, the orthopaedic resident took a careful medical history before examining her and learned that she had had a mastectomy five years earlier but otherwise had had no serious medical problems. Unfortunately, the roentgenogram of the femur showed a large lucent lesion with a pathologic fracture that was most likely a metastatic focus related to her mastectomy. Many complex biochemical and biological activities are associated with such a fracture, but some are straightforward biomechanical ones, and the question arises, "How does replacement of bone by tumor weaken the bone?"

In this chapter we use the basic concepts developed earlier to analyze the effect of pathological conditions on the strength of bone and its propensity to fracture. Let us review several concepts important in this analysis.

■ 9.1 FRACTURES

A variety of loading conditions can be experienced by the bone of the musculoskeletal system. These include tension/compression, bending, shear, torsion, and complex combinations of these conditions. The forces responsible for these modes of loading may be internal (due to muscle action) or external (due to contact with objects extrinsic to the body). The forces that produce fractures are almost always of the second type, for example, contact with the ground at the end of a fall. Exceptions to the general rule are more likely to occur, however, if pathologic bone is involved. For example, muscle forces and gravity (against which the muscles must react) are often the only sources of loading present when osteoporotic bone fails (as in hip fractures or crushing of vertebral bodies in the elderly).

Strength also refers to the stress at fracture, and the strength of compact bone depends strongly on the direction in which the stress acts relative to the axis of the bone. This directional dependence of strength is called *anisotropy,* and we will see in chapter 17 that anisotropy is a consequence of the internal (osteonal) structure of bone at the microscopic level. At the macroscopic level, compact bone is strongest in compression, intermediate in tension, and weakest in shear or torsion (figure 9.1). Under the complex loading that occurs during trauma, however,

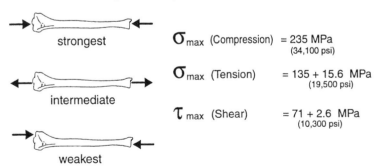

strongest

intermediate

weakest

σ_{max} (Compression) = 235 MPa
(34,100 psi)

σ_{max} (Tension) = 135 + 15.6 MPa
(19,500 psi)

τ_{max} (Shear) = 71 + 2.6 MPa
(10,300 psi)

Figure 9.1. Bone is anisotropic and displays different material properties in different directions. For long bones in the longitudinal direction, cortical bone is strongest in compression, intermediate in tension, and weakest in shear. *Adapted from:* Cochran GVB: *A Primer of Orthopaedic Biomechanics.* Churchill Livingstone, New York, 1982, p. 161. *Data adapted from:* Reilly DT, Burstein AH: The elastic and ultimate properties of compact bone tissue. *J Biomechanics* 8:393, 1975.

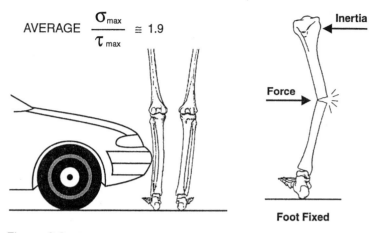

$$\text{AVERAGE } \frac{\sigma_{max}}{\tau_{max}} \cong 1.9$$

Inertia

Force

Foot Fixed

Figure 9.2. Bending is the most common mode of loading for most injuries, as illustrated by this schematic of a car hitting a human being.

combinations of these "pure" stresses are usually generated. Fractures with different geometries result from the interplay of these combined stresses with the anisotropic properties of the bone. Bending is the most commonly encountered mode of loading during trauma (figure 9.2). Pure bending produces transverse fractures (tension of the convex side of the bone). In pure torsion, we have seen that spiral fractures are produced. Pure tension is essentially impossible to impose on a bone other than in the laboratory and is never encountered clinically. Compression, or crushing, does occur, and pure compression will produce a shear failure at 45° to the compression axis. Combined loading, such as bending and torsion of the tibia, in a fall are the general rule and lead to fractures with various degrees of obliquity.

Another important consideration in bone fracture is the amount of energy absorbed by the tissue. As the velocity of impact increases, the (kinetic) energy of the encounter increases as the square of the velocity. At low velocities, enough energy is available to create only the fracture surfaces described (figure 9.3). If more energy is delivered, displacement of the fragments will occur. At even higher velocities, ample energy will be available to generate multiple fracture surfaces, and comminuted fractures will result. Consider the difference in tissue disruption and fracture pattern of a high-velocity gunshot wound or a twisting fracture of the tibia caused by a slip on a wet floor (figure 9.4).

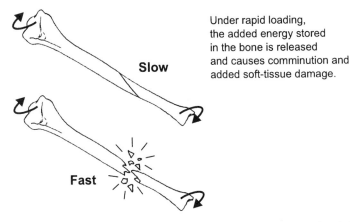

Under rapid loading, the added energy stored in the bone is released and causes comminution and added soft-tissue damage.

Figure 9.3. The rate of loading effects the type of fracture and soft tissue injury. *Source:* Cochran GVB: *A Primer of Orthopaedic Biomechanics.* Churchill Livingstone, New York, 1982, p. 171.

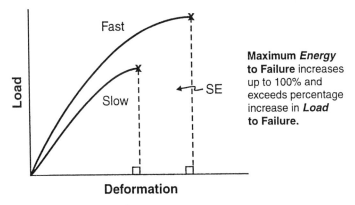

Maximum *Energy* to Failure increases up to 100% and exceeds percentage increase in ***Load* to Failure.**

Figure 9.4. The rate of loading of a bone also affects its load to failure and the energy to failure. The representative data shown in this graph are for failure of cortical bone in the transverse plane. *Source:* Cochran GVB: *A Primer of Orthopaedic Biomechanics.* Churchill Livingstone, New York, 1982, p. 170.

■ 9.2 FRACTURE IN ABNORMAL BONE

Even though forces in the fracture situation described in Section 9.1 are transmitted through skin, muscle, and other soft tissues, we consider these types of situations as examples of damage created by direct forces through either bending, torsion, or compression. Fractured bones may also be created by indirect forces—such as excessive muscle pull on a bone (perhaps transmitted via the tendon)—creating *tensile* forces in the bone. A perfect example is transverse fracture of the patella associated with sudden knee flexion and quadriceps muscle contraction (figure 9.5).

All of the preceding concepts have been explored more extensively in chapters 3, 4, 5, 7, and 8 but are summarized here to help us understand what happens when there is a deficit in a bone. Actually, one of the more common presentations of malignant disease in bone, be it primary (as in multiple myeloma) or secondary (as in metastatic cancer) is a type of fracture that can be thought of as an insufficiency fracture occurring in weakened bone (figure 9.6). Pathologic fractures can usually be identified by history, examination, and roentgenographic appearance; evaluation of a patient with such a problem is centered on discovering the reason for the patient's weakened bone. Bone is weakened as a tumor grows, for example, and there are fewer and fewer supporting cancellous trabecular pillars to support body weight and withstand the bending moments associated with nearly constant spinal move-

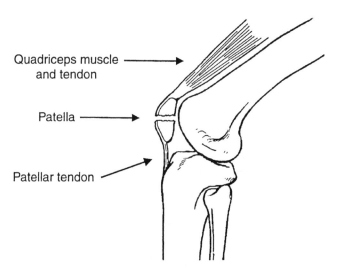

Figure 9.5. This transverse fracture of a patella is an example of an indirect force, such as the pull (transmitted by the tendons) of a muscle on a bone, creating tensile stress in the bone.

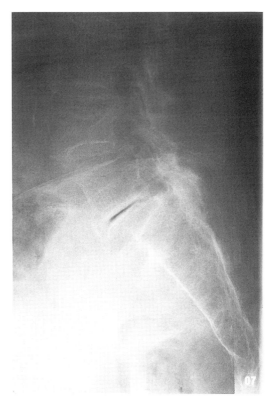

Figure 9.6. Roentgeneogram of a compression fracture in a patient with osteoporosis.

ments. Nonneoplastic weakening of vertebrae, as seen in osteoporosis (figure 9.6), creates similar problems with structural integrity of the vertebrae. The strength of a vertebral body can be measured directly only in cadaveric specimens but can be indirectly ascertained by several means. Plain roentgenograms, quantitative CT scans, or photon density studies all give important information relating to vertebral integrity. Figure 9.7 depicts an example of an experimental study illustrating the strength/density relationship.

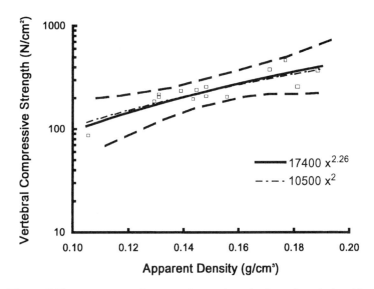

Figure 9.7. The results of an experimental study show the relationship between the density of the cancellous bone and the compressive strength of the vertebrae. *Source: Orthopaedic Science: A Resource and Self-Study Guide for the Practitioner.* American Academy of Orthopaedic Surgeons, Rosemont, Ill., 1986, chapter 5, slide v-50, p. 171.

Compression fractures are most common in cancellous bone, but cortical bone can also be compressed to failure. Figure 9.8 indicates that such failure occurs at 45° to the load axis. A somewhat similar mode of failure occurs in shear loading in certain situations, such as in a tibial plateau fracture where there is a load applied parallel to the articular surface, shearing off the tibial plateau.

■ 9.3 BONE WEAKENING

Bone affected by more obvious pathological processes becomes weakened through a variety of enzymatic, chemical, and cellular changes that ultimately result in osteoclastic activity and bone loss. Osteoclast precursors are present in bone, circulate in the bloodstream, and are attracted to sites of bone resorption associated with systemic disorders

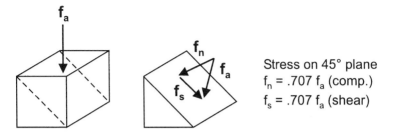

Stress on 45° plane
f_n = .707 f_a (comp.)
f_s = .707 f_a (shear)

Pure compressive loading on cortical bone leads to
shear failure at 45° to the load axis.

Figure 9.8. Cortical bone fails in shear at the 45° plane under compressive loading.

such as hyperparathyroidism or primary or secondary tumors. Resorption of bone at such sites is due to an increase in both the number and activity of osteoclasts. The osteoclast is the final pathway for bone resorption, a process modified by the presence of osteoblasts, stromal cells, cytokines (particularly interleukin-6), prostoglandins, and other local factors. Only in the late stages of tumor infiltration does the tumor itself destroy bone by a combination of enzymatic and cellular processes. Such defects may be small, but they constitute stress concentrations or stress risers. Even a screw hole acts as a stress riser, but any small hole in the bone will decrease bending strength by 50% or energy absorption by 75% (figures 9.9a and b). Larger holes are called open-section defects. An open-section defect also weakens the bone, but to a greater extent— torque resistance decreases by 70%, and energy absorption decreases up to 90% for large open-section defects. Another way to appreciate the effect of size of a metastatic defect is to review figure 9.10, which shows progressive strength reduction as the hole diameter/bone diameter ratio increases (i.e., the open-section defect enlarges).

Thus it is obvious that any loss of bone substance will subject a particular bone to increased risk of fracture and create the terrible problem that haunts patients with malignant disease. A significant clinical challenge is to identify when the probability of pathological fracture has increased to the point where prophylactic stabilization is warranted; precise methods of determining this, however, have not been developed.

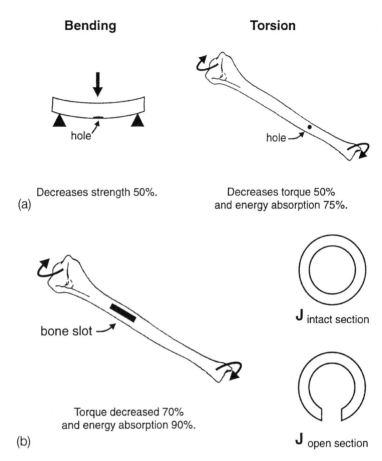

Bending

Torsion

hole

hole

Decreases strength 50%.

(a)

Decreases torque 50%
and energy absorption 75%.

bone slot

J intact section

Torque decreased 70%
and energy absorption 90%.

(b)

J open section

Figure 9.9. *(a)* Long bones are weakened (that is, load-to-failure is decreased, and energy absorption is reduced) in both bending and torsion when hole defects are present. *Source:* Cochran GVB: *A Primer of Orthopaedic Biomechanics.* Churchill Livingstone, New York, 1982, p. 165. *(b)* An open-section defect also reduces the torque to failure and energy-absorption capability of a long bone. The polar moment of inertia of the slotted section is greatly reduced when compared to the intact section. *Source:* Cochran GVB: *A Primer of Orthopaedic Biomechanics.* Churchill Livingstone, New York, 1982, p. 167.

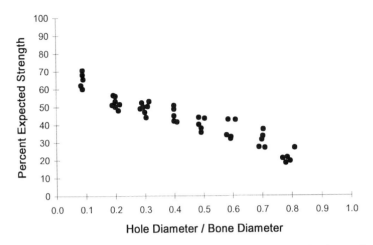

Figure 9.10. As the ratio of the size of a hole defect to the bone diameter increases, the strength of the bone decreases. *Source: Orthopaedic Science: A Resource and Self-Study Guide for the Practitioner.* American Academy of Orthopaedic Surgeons, Rosemont, Ill., 1986, chapter 5, slide v-52, p. 172.

The most widely quoted parameters for predicting probability of a fracture through a metastatic lesion in the femur are those supplied by Harrington. These are 1) a lesion 2.5 cm or greater, 2) lytic destruction of greater than 50% of the bone's circumference, and 3) persistent pain with weight bearing despite local radiotherapy. A pathologic fracture often occurs when the patient is not in optimum condition, leading to significant pain and hospitalization. Recognition of impending fracture and prophylactic bony stabilization may allow surgery to be carried out when the patient is better able to tolerate such surgery (figure 9.11). Thus we see that Matilda sustained a pathologic fracture of her femur because the metastasis in the bone had created a large-section defect and substantially weakened the bone.

Q9: CLINICAL QUESTION (SUMMARY)

Matilda's roentgenogram of her broken femur showed a large lucent lesion with a pathologic fracture that was most likely a

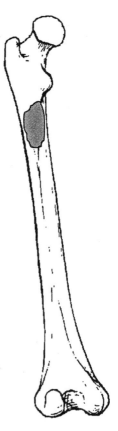

Figure 9.11. Lytic lesions in a proximal femur, like the one in Matilda's femur, substantially weaken the bone structure.

metastatic focus related to her mastectomy. How did the replacement of bone by the tumor weaken the bone?

A9: CLINICAL ANSWER

Matilda sustained a pathologic fracture of her femur because the metastasis in the bone had created a large-section defect, which substantially weakened the bone. This answer is given in detail in Section 9.3.

Additional Reading

Athanasou NA: Cellular Biology of Bone-Resorbing Cells. *J Bone Joint Surg* 78A:1096–1107, 1996.

Frankel VH, Burnstein AH: *Orthopaedic Biomechanics,* 1st ed. Lea and Febiger, Philadelphia, 1970.

Harrington KD: New Trends in the Management of Lower Extremity Metastases. *Clin Orthop* 169:53–61, 1982.

Pugh J, Sherry HS, Futterman B, Frankel VH: Biomechanics of Pathologic Fractures. *Clin Orthop* 169:109–114, 1982.

10

Mechanics of Treatment

CLINICAL SCENARIO: EXTERNAL FIXATION AND FRACTURE HEALING

Charley Davidson did not belong to a motorcycle gang. He had never heard of Sturgis, South Dakota, and did not even have a tattoo, but he loved the rush of wind in his face as he rode his big motorcycle back and forth to work. He was a very careful rider and always wore his helmet, but he was always worried about the lack of courtesy automobile drivers often show around bikes. It was not discourtesy, however, that caused a pickup truck suddenly to turn in front of him. The ensuing collision with a road sign resulted in a severe, open fracture of Davidson's leg. After an assessment in the emergency room indicated no other injuries, he was taken to the operating room, where the large soft tissue wound was cleaned and debrided, and his tibia stabilized with a monoplane external fixture. Will such a stabilization device allow this fracture to heal?

The many choices for treatment of fractures—bone plates, intramedullary (IM) nails, external fixators—seem overwhelming at times. The rationale for use of the various devices is somewhat vague and nonspecific in many cases even though entire books are written on the subject of specific fracture-fixation techniques. In this chapter, we cover only the basic biomechanical concepts of screws, bone plates, external fixators, and intramedullary rods. Other aspects of fracture treatment are best found in other sources.

■ 10.1 BIOMECHANICAL REQUIREMENTS FOR FRACTURE HEALING

Direct apposition, rigid fixation, and axial compression provide optimal conditions for healing of fracture-generated gaps in a bone. The size of the gap and the presence or absence of motion will govern the type of tissue that forms within it. Figure 10.1 shows an exaggerated

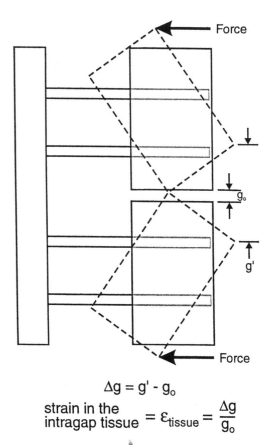

$$\Delta g = g' - g_o$$

$$\text{strain in the intragap tissue} = \varepsilon_{tissue} = \frac{\Delta g}{g_o}$$

Figure 10.1. In this exaggerated picture of a bone stabilized with an external fixator, the fracture gap opening has a strain of $\Delta g/g_o$. The original size of the gap and the displacement will determine the strain in (and therefore the type of) the tissue that forms in the gap.

schematic of a typical fracture with a gap opening due to an applied force. The strain across the gap is equal to the change in gap opening normalized to the original gap size. As a general rule of thumb, for a given gap size, strains between 10% and 100% will cause granulation tissue to form, strains of 2% to 10% produce fibrocartilage, and strains of less than 2% result in bone filling in the gap. In fracture gaps with strains of greater than 10%, the granulation tissue that forms helps to stabilize the gap and reduce the strain, enabling either fibrocartilage or bone eventually to form. If the strain exceeds the strength of the in-growing tissue, damage will occur, and a pseudoarthrosis may form. The goal of fracture treatment is therefore to align the components as accurately as possible and fix them together rigidly to control the intra-gap motion so that the bone can heal with bone (that is, mineralized tissue) without intervening steps. Any technique used to stabilize a fracture should have a fixation rigidity in the range of 20%–60% of the intact bone in bending.

■ 10.2 BIOMECHANICS OF BONE SCREWS

Bone screws are the most commonly used type of orthopaedic implant. Just as there are different screws used for attaching metal components (machine screws) and wood parts (wood screws), so there are different screw types used for cortical bone and cancellous bone. Some simple terms are used to describe screws. Proper use of these terms helps to facilitate understanding of how the different screws function.

Figure 10.2 shows the basic anatomy of a screw. The screw has two diameters: the *root diameter* and the *outer diameter*. The root diameter refers to the minimum diameter of the screw across the base of the threads. The area defined by the section of the root diameter is called the *root area*. The root area governs the maximum tensile and shear loads that can be applied to the screw. The outer diameter of the screw is the distance across the maximum thread width. The *pitch* of a screw is the distance between threads. For example, a screw with 10 threads per inch has a pitch of 1/10 inch. In simple screws with only one thread, the *lead* (or the distance a screw advances with one revolution) equals the pitch.

Screws function by converting the insertion torque into internal tension in the screw and into elastic reactions in the surrounding material, which creates compression of the components the screw holds together. The huge difference in material properties of cortical and cancellous

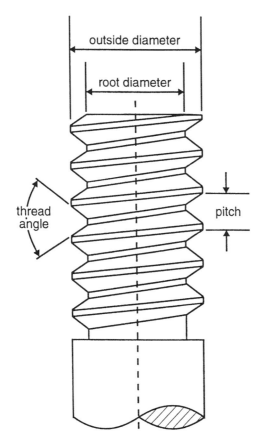

Figure 10.2. A schematic of a typical screw thread with several of the parameters that are used to describe a screw. *Source:* Perren SM, Cordey J, Baumgart F, Rahn BA, Schatzker J: Technical and biomechanical aspects of screws used for bone surgery. *Inter J. of Ortho Trauma* 2:31–48, 1992.

bone makes the elastic reaction around the screw very different. This concept is critical in understanding the differences between cortical and cancellous screws and their holding power in bone.

10.2.1 Cortical Bone Screws

Cortical bone screws are similar to machine screws in function and design. For machine screws, a hole of a diameter equal to the root diameter of the screw is predrilled. The hole is then tapped to form the threads into which the screw is threaded. Self-tapping cortical bone screws have the cutting head of the tap milled into the tip of the screw, thus requiring no separate tapping operation.

> ➤ Cortical bone screws are similar to machine screws.

The torque used to drive a screw can be large because of the moment arm of the grip surface of the screwdriver. For this reason, screws should be inserted with care. Shearing failure and thread failure of the cortical screw during insertion is not uncommon. It occurs because the pilot hole is too small, the screw is incorrectly aligned in the hole, or because the torques required to cut the threads during insertion are so large. As the thickness of the cortical wall increases, the torque required to drive the screw also increases, thus putting the screw in more jeopardy. In addition, if the pilot hole for self-tapping screws is too small, the torque for insertion will be very high. However, if the pilot hole is too large, screw purchase will be reduced.

As mentioned previously, the shear strength of the screw is related to the root diameter. For a screw with a given outer diameter, deep threads will give good purchase in the bone, but they will also lessen the screw's resistance to shear. Increasing the root diameter of the screw even slightly will greatly increase its strength and stiffness (see chapter 5). By trial and error, cortical bone screws have been developed with relatively large root diameters and shallow threads. This combination has been found to give the best tradeoff of screw strength versus purchase in the bone.

When machine screws are used in metal parts, the screw will more than likely fail first when being extracted. The opposite is true for cortical bone screws because the stiffness and strength of the bone is so much less than that of the metal screws. The resistance of a cortical screw to pullout depends on the shear strength of the bone into which it is embedded, its depth of insertion into the bone, and the outer diameter of the screw, which determines the amount of bone within the threads. Of these factors in a properly placed cortical screw, the outer diameter of the screw is the most important.

10.2.2 Cancellous Bone Screws

Cancellous bone screws are similar to wood screws in design and function. They have large, deep threads that grip the spongy bone well. Failure of cancellous bone screws during insertion is much less of a problem than with cortical screws because the bone is not as strong, and friction is lower. The parameters that governed the resistance of a cortical screw to extraction also govern the pullout of the cancellous bone screw, but, because the cancellous bone is weaker, the threads must be deeper. In addition, the density of the bone is now very important. Higher-density cancellous bone is stronger and will increase the pullout strength of the screw in the bone.

➢ Cancellous bone screws are similar to wood screws.

For cancellous screws, purchase of the screw into the bone is very important. For that reason, the size of the pilot hole should be about the size of the root diameter, and oversized holes should be avoided. In addition, studies have shown that tapping the hole before insertion is detrimental to the pullout strength of the screw in cancellous bone.

■ 10.3 BIOMECHANICS OF BONE PLATES

A bone plate is essentially an internal splint that holds the fracture fragments together. The functions of a bone plate are to maintain alignment, prevent relative motion, and, if possible, create compression between the ends of the fracture or neutralize forces created across the fracture site. If compression is achieved, load is transferred to the bone and not carried solely by the plate. Bone plates are not designed to carry all the load originally carried by the bone.

Dynamic-compression (DC) bone plates are specifically designed to bring the ends of a bone fracture together and to compress them. The DC plate has a special type of hole on one or both sides of the plate. This hole is elongated with an inclined surface (shown schematically in figure 10.3). As the bone screw is inserted with torque, it moves down

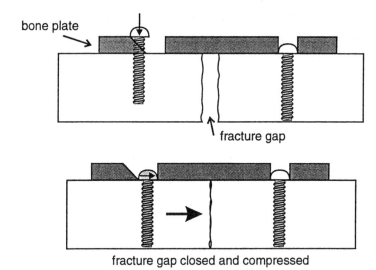

bone plate

fracture gap

fracture gap closed and compressed

Figure 10.3. The dynamic-compression plate is designed with an incline on which the screw slides as it is inserted. The screw (with the bone attached) slides so as to close the fracture gap and provide compression across the fracture site.

the incline. This forces the bone screw (and therefore the attached bone) to move toward the center of the plate. The fractured ends are thus brought into contact and compressed.

In many cases, the bones of the body are loaded in bending, which puts one side under tension and the opposite side under compression. If the bone plate is placed on the tension side, it will help resist opening of the gap, and the plate itself will be shielded from carrying the whole load. Figure 10.4 illustrates this concept. If the plate is placed (incorrectly) on the compression side, the gap opening will be greater under the influence of an applied bending moment because the bone in the vicinity of the fracture carries none of the load. Furthermore, the plate will experience higher stresses because it alone must resist the bending moment. This increases the likelihood of its early failure by fatigue. There are cases in the body when the locations of tension and compression vary throughout an activity cycle, for example, in gait. The best that can be done in these cases is to ensure initial compression across the fracture site.

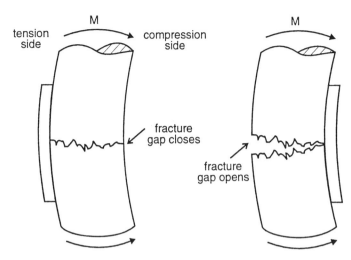

Figure 10.4. If a bone plate is placed on the tension side of the fracture, the bone can contribute to resisting an applied bending moment through compression of the fracture surfaces. Conversely, if the bone plate is placed on the compression side of the bone, the plate has to carry the majority of the load, and the fracture site is in tension and opens. *Source:* Tencer AF, Johnson KD: *Biomechanics in Orthopaedic Trauma-Bone Fracture and Fixation.* JB Lippincott Company, Philadelphia, 1994, p. 148, figure 6.43.

10.3.1 Permanent Deformation in Bending of Bone Plates

Bone plates are often bent to conform to the shape of the bone. Bending of the plate is essential to provide maximum friction of the plate against the bone. However, plastic (or permanent) deformation of the plate reduces the amount of strain energy that the plate can absorb and makes it more susceptible to fatigue failure. For that reason, bone plates are usually made of materials with high ductility (specifically, certain grades of stainless steel) that can absorb enormous amounts of deformation without being totally compromised. This subject is discussed in greater depth in chapter 14.

10.3.2 Bending Rigidity of Bone Plates

Although high-rigidity bone plates provide rigid fixation for fracture healing, they can also shield the bone from stress. In chapter 6 we discussed the problems of stress shielding by bone plates. Bone plates must be stiff enough to allow for fracture healing yet flexible to reduce the effects of stress shielding. Bone plates are sometimes removed after the fracture has healed in order to reduce bone resorption. Various investigators have proposed the use of composite plates or absorbable composite plates; however, there are many technical problems with such devices, and to date no such device is on the market.

■ 10.4 BIOMECHANICS OF EXTERNAL FIXATION

Of the many different general types of external fixation, the most commonly used fixators can be categorized into five classifications: 1) unilateral, 2) bilateral, 3) triangular, 4) quadrilateral, and 5) closed or semicircular ring configurations. Because healing of the fracture is controlled in part by reducing gap opening at the fracture site, the key biomechanical factor in judging the performance of an external fixator is the bone-segment rigidity after fixation. (The concepts of rigidity in bending and torsion were discussed at length in chapters 4 and 5.) Many experimental tests have determined the rigidity of these different configurations; chapter 12 discusses how these types of tests might be performed.

These are the main parameters that might effect bone-segment rigidity.

- Number of pins
- Pin diameter
- Connecting-rod (side-bar) separation
- Pin separation within a group
- Distance from pin group to fracture site
- Half-pin or full-pin configuration
- Number of connecting rods
- Symmetry (or asymmetry) of the connecting-rod application
- Pin and frame material
- Compression at the fracture site
- Type of fracture

Of these many parameters, studies show that to increase the rigidity of an external fixator most effectively, one can do the following:

- Increase the number of pins
- Increase the pin diameter
- Decrease pin length (or decrease side-bar separation)
- Use multiplane pin fixation (to increase both bending and torsional rigidity) or increase the number of connecting rods
- Induce compression across the fracture site.

Increasing the number of pins increases fixation rigidity by increasing the system's area and polar moments of inertia; however, studies demonstrate that, in general, the increase becomes less significant when more than eight pins are used.

Increasing pin diameter by a slight amount can make a big difference in frame rigidity because the pin's area moment of inertia (which actually controls rigidity) depends on the pin diameter raised to the *fourth power*. However, increasing pin diameter also increases the stress-concentration effects in the bone, which may cause bone necrosis or fracture at the pin-insertion site.

The length of the pins controls the magnitude of the maximum moment (or torque), which bends the rods and produces fracture gap opening. Decreasing the length of the pins decreases this moment as a first-order effect.

Unilateral half-pin frames are significantly lower in rigidity (especially torsional rigidity) than the bilateral full-pin frames. Increasing the number of connecting rods increases the torsional and bending rigidity as well. However, increasing the number of components also limits exposure of soft tissue and is not always possible.

Compression across the fracture site by prestressing the pins cannot always be achieved but does add stability to the system. However, excessive compression can overload the pins and lead to permanent pin deformation and possible failure in fatigue. Maximum stresses in the pin occur at the pin-bone junction. Permanently deformed pins are not an uncommon clinical finding; they can lead to loss of fracture reduction and difficulty in pin removal.

■ 10.5 BIOMECHANICS OF INTRAMEDULLARY NAILS

Intramedullary (IM) nails also act as internal splints for a fracture. Just as with other fracture fixation devices, the likelihood of bone healing with an IM nail depends in part on the rigidity and stability of the fixation. IM nails hold the fracture together by providing axial alignment and allow limited motion of the stable fracture site. Torsional rigidity of the IM nail in the bone depends on the size and shape of the rod and the friction of the nail in the IM canal. Newer versions of IM nails have insertion of perpendicular "locking" screws that add increased rotational stability (see Section 10.5.1). The canal is reamed to improve the fit between the bone and the nail. Fractures best fixed with the standard IM nail are those that exhibit good inherent torsional rigidity around the midshaft.

When an intramedullary rod is in place in the bone, fracture gap opening due to bending is controlled by the bending rigidity of the nail and the stability of the fracture site. At first it may seem that the more rigid the nail, the better. However, there is more to consider than just fracture-fixation rigidity. Insertion of the nail down the IM canal of a slightly curved bone can be tricky. A more flexible nail is easier to insert into the canal and reduces the risk of splitting the canal due to the hoop (or circumferential) stresses created during insertion into a slightly undersized canal. Slotted nails have decreased rigidity yet still allow fracture healing in many cases. A disadvantage of the slotted nail is that it is substantially weaker than the unslotted nail and is therefore more susceptible to failure in fatigue. Although relatively rare, cracks and fractures of slotted nails have been reported.

10.5.1 Interlocked IM Nails

Standard IM nails that are locked with a screw on the proximal end act only as internal gliding splints of fractures. They allow no resistance to shortening of comminuted fractures. Interlocking the device with screws at both ends of the nail across the fracture site gives the bone axial support. Interlocking of the nail with limited or no support at the fracture site forces the nail to carry more of the load and leaves it more susceptible to failure in fatigue.

10.5.1.1 Dynamization of Interlocked IM Nail

After the fracture has partially healed, the interlocked intramedullary nail still supports much of the load. Compressive loading of the partially healed fracture site may stimulate better bone quality and faster healing while reducing the effects of stress shielding. Dynamization of the interlocked nail is accomplished by removing the distal screws. Dynamization also reduces stress in the nail and reduces its risk of fatigue fracture.

Q10: Clinical Question (Summary)

Charley Davidson loved his motorcycle, but he did not love the pickup truck with which he collided. He sustained an open fracture of his tibia with large soft tissue involvement that was stabilized with a monoplane external fixator. Will such a stabilization device allow this fracture to heal?

A10: Clinical Answer

Fracture stabilization is a race between bone healing and the longevity of the fixation device. Fortunately, the bone usually wins but not always. A fixation device must be rigid to provide stabilization of the fracture; if too much flexibility is allowed in the system, the bone ends may form a pseudoarthrosis instead of normal bone healing. In addition, in the external fixator system, too much flexibility means increased stresses in the pins, which can result in pin bending or fatigue failure. As discussed in Section 10.4, the use of multiplane external fixator configurations are effective in increasing the rigidity of an external fixator. The monoplane external fixator may indeed allow the fracture to heal, but a multiplane fixator would have been a better choice of treatment of Mr. Davidson's fracture.

Additional Reading

Chao EYS, Aro HT: Biomechanics of fracture fixation. In *Basic Orthopaedic Biomechanics,* VC Mow, WC Hayes, Eds. Raven Press, New York, 1991.

Current Concepts of Internal Fixation of Fractures, HK Uhthoff, Ed. Springer-Verlag, Berlin, 1980.

Jennings J, Kirkpatrick L, Mukherjee A: Cable-Ready Cable Grip System Bone Plate. Technical Monograph 97–2232–06. Zimmer, Inc., Warsaw, Ind., 1997.

Science and Practice of Intramedullary Nailing, BD Browner, CC Edwards, Eds. Lea & Febiger, Philadelphia, 1987.

Tencer AF, Johnson KD: *Biomechanics in Orthopedic Trauma—Bone Fracture and Fixation.* JB Lippincott Co., Philadelphia, 1994.

11

Mechanics of Implants

CLINICAL SCENARIO: FRACTURE OF AN INTRAMEDULLARY ROD

Charley Davidson's pal Sanza Time had a similar accident, but, instead of fracturing his tibia, he sustained a closed fracture of the femur. This fracture was treated by closed intramedullary rodding, and Sanza, against the advice of his surgeon, was back on his bike as soon as the repair shop pronounced it ready. Also against the advice of his doctor, he went back to his job in a steel mill, where he was on his feet all day, and even played a little softball on weekends. His doctor was hardly surprised, then, that, about 11 weeks after his operation, Sanza had a sudden pain in the thigh. A roentgenogram showed a broken rod associated with an ununited femur. How could such a thing happen?

The hip bone's connected to the thigh bone. The thigh bone's connected to the total knee arthroplasty ... Whoops! That's not how the saying is supposed to go. In the current days of orthopaedics, however, such is often the case. Orthopaedic implants have given many people back the freedom to perform everyday activities. One fundamental aspect of all types of implants is that they transmit load to the biological structure. In this chapter, we discuss these load-transmission mechanisms and pull together ideas presented in other chapters to present an overall picture of the basic concepts of the mechanics of implants.

■ 11.1 LOAD SHARING VERSUS LOAD TRANSFER

Implants are generally categorized as load-sharing or load-transferring devices. A load-sharing implant is one in which the implant may carry all the load part of the time but shares the load with the bone at least some of the time. An example of a load-sharing implant is a bone plate: The plate may carry all the load for an unstable fracture across the section of the instability, but it shares the load where it is attached to the bone. Load-transferring implants, on the other hand, transfer load only from one bony part to another. An example of a load-transferring implant is a total knee replacement, where the device transfers the joint reaction force from the sectioned femoral condyle to the cut surface of the tibia. The mechanics of these two types of devices play an important role in their design, performance, and clinical use.

11.1.1 Load-Sharing Implants

The rigidity of the load-sharing implant controls how much load the implant shares with the surrounding bone. (This concept was discussed in detail in chapter 6) In most cases, the bending rigidity of the implant is the most important factor in determining how much load is shared with the bone. The rigidity of an implant is a function of both the size and shape of the implant (I) and the material stiffness (E).

➤ Load-sharing implants share the load with the bone at least part of the time.

11.1.1.1 The Race between Healing and Device Failure

Most load-sharing implants are not (or cannot be) designed to carry all the load applied to the bone indefinitely. Ideally, when a well-fixed load-sharing implant is in place in the bone, the fracture heals, or the interface stabilizes, and the implant does not have to carry all the load across an unstable fracture site for very long. What happens, however, when an implant has to support all the load in the bone for a longer-than-expected period of time? Examples of this situation are 1) an intramedullary rod stabilizing a fracture that goes to nonunion or 2) the femoral component of a total hip replacement in which the proximal femur experiences severe osteolysis due to stress shielding and particle disease. In such cases, the implant is subjected to higher stresses or longer periods of loading than were anticipated in its design, and the implant is thus at risk of failure due to fatigue. (The concepts of fatigue failure were discussed in detail in chapter 8.) Other forms of clinical failure of the implant, such as instability, loosening, breaking of the cement mantle, and so on, may also occur. Especially in the case of fracture fixation, there is always a race between implant failure and healing.

11.1.2 Load-Transferring Implants

Load-transferring implants transfer load between the implant and the adjoining structure, usually the epiphysis of a long bone or the surface of a joint. In this type of implant, the entire load is carried by the device, and these implants are often subjected to high joint reaction forces. Examples of load-transferring implants are tibial plateaus in total knee replacement and acetabular components in total hip replacements.

> ➤ Load-transferring implants carry the entire load.

When considering load-transferring implants, one must take into account several mechanical factors that relate to how the load is distributed to the bone and through the interface between the implant and bone. If stresses in the contacting bone are localized and very high, fatigue failure of that region is likely; at the same time, stress shielding and bone resorption of the other regions can be predicted. Likewise, if the distribution of stress to the bone is adequate, but the stresses at the prosthesis-bone interface are very high, then the interface—whether it be fixation by tissue ingrowth or cement—is prone to failure.

Deformation of and stresses in the implant must also be considered. The implant design must ensure that the elastic deformation that occurs with loading does not lead to early implant failure or to changes in the load distribution to the bone and interface. In total knee arthroplasty, the thin all-polyethylene tibial component that was used at one time is an example of failure to consider this concept. The implant design seemed adequate until one considered the deformation of the implant in the body under constant load for an extended period of time. Polyethylene is a viscoelastic material and is subject to creep (or cold flow). Cold flow in polymers is the gradually increasing deformation produced by long-term loading (see chapters 16 and 17). These implants became distorted, changed the path of load transfer to the tibia, and often fractured. A classic study by Bartel et al. used finite-element modeling to determine stresses in polyethylene tibial trays. The results of this analysis showed that a metal backing should be used on conventional flat polyethylene tibial-bearing surface designs and that the thickness of the polyethylene should be at least 8 mm.

■ 11.2 FINITE ELEMENT MODELING AND ANALYSIS IN ORTHOPAEDICS

Finite element modeling (FEM) is an engineering analysis tool that is often used to assist in the design of implants and devices. In finite element modeling, a geometric representation, or model, of the part in question is formed by using many building blocks called elements. These elements are of finite, or given, size (thus the term *finite element modeling*). When a three-dimensional (3-D) model is made, the elements can be of various shapes, such as bricks (fairly regular six-sided solids) and tetrahedrons (four-sided solids); in two-dimensional (2-D) models, the elements are usually quadrilaterals and triangles. Additional elements (such as beams, spars, shells, and plates) are also available for use in both 2-D and 3-D modeling.

To form a model, many elements are joined to form the approximate shape of the part. The collection of elements is referred to as a *mesh.* The elements fit together to fill space. The corners where a number of elements meet are referred to as *nodes.* Each of these elements is assigned its own material properties that represent the properties of the part in the location of the element. For example, in modeling the proximal femur, cortical-bone properties would be assigned to the elements of the midshaft, whereas cancellous-bone properties would be assigned to the elements at the center of the femoral head.

One can conceive of a finite element model as a kind of free-body diagram of a structure in which each individual element that contributes to the model must obey the rules of static equilibrium. Once the model is formed, the boundary conditions (or outside constraints) are set according to what happens in real life. For example, if the femur in one-legged stance is being modeled, then the condyles would have to be restrained from moving by applying nondisplacement criteria on the nodes at the distal end of the model. Forces are also applied to the model at the nodes that represent points where forces act on the real structure. These forces can be applied as either single quantities or distributed loads. More sophisticated modeling techniques (for example, contact elements that allow sliding with or without friction, nonlinear material properties, etc.) are also available.

When all parameters are set, the finite element computer program is directed to solve the problem. It does this by looking at constitutive equations for each element individually and then linking them to solve simultaneously. Constitutive equations are an engineering term for the relationship between load and displacement (and therefore stress and strain). It is not hard to solve for stress and strain in just one simple element. However, solving thousands of equations all at the same time (for even a relatively simple model) is essentially impossible without the use of a computer. It is easy to see why increasing the number of elements in a model increases both the complexity of the solution and the time (and computing hardware) required to analyze it.

The output of finite element models is usually presented in the form of stress maps. These maps yield important information about the distribution of stress throughout the structure. Many times, displacement plots also provide useful information. Specific values of stress, strain, displacement, and force at any node in the model can also be obtained. This information is extremely important for predicting how implants will function in the body.

11.2.1 Special Considerations in Finite Element Modeling

True or false?: Every stress and strain result obtained from a finite element analysis is the correct answer for the part being modeled. The answer is False! Just because the computer spits out a solution does not mean that it is correct for the real-life situation. The problem is not with the computer, however, but with the way in which the model was formed. The results of any finite element analysis are only as good as the model from which they were obtained. In considering the validity of FEM results, we must examine many factors.

11.2.1.1 Convergence

Consider a three-dimensional, finite element model of a sphere. Figure 11.1a shows a sphere that was modeled using 23 four-sided shell elements. Clearly, 23 elements are not sufficient to represent the true shape of the sphere. Figure 11.1b shows a model of a sphere using 253 elements; this model would predict stresses much more accurately than the one using only 23 elements.

Now consider this same concept applied to a complicated part. The more elements a model has, the better it should predict stresses. *Convergence* is the term used to describe the situation that exists when an adequate number of elements has been used in the model, leading to consistent results. If the number of elements in a given model is increased, and the stress result changes significantly, the model has not reached convergence and must undergo further mesh refinement (i.e., more elements must be added). Adding more elements, however, dramatically increases the complexity of the problem. In order to obtain good results yet minimize the number of elements, localized mesh refinement is often done. In this way, only the areas of complex geometry (or the areas where a knowledge of stress magnitudes is important) need to have detailed meshes. Figure 11.2 illustrates this concept. In this model of the condyle of a femoral knee component with a patellar

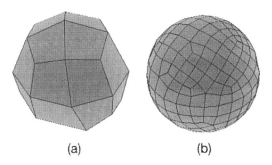

(a)   (b)

Figure 11.1. A finite element mesh of a sphere using 23 four-sided shell elements (a) is a very rough approximation of the true shape. When 253 elements are employed (b), the mesh is a much better representation of a sphere.

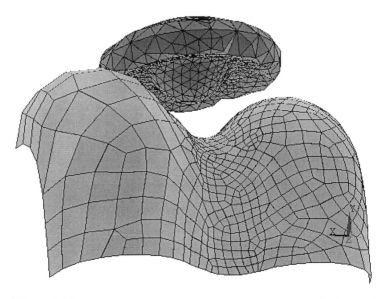

Figure 11.2. A finite element mesh model of the condyle of a femoral knee component with a patellar button.

button, the edges of the patellar button are not of great concern. They can be modeled coarsely, whereas the middle back of the button and the condylar notch are more detailed.

11.2.1.2 Limitations of Finite Element Models

When biological structures are modeled, it is important to keep in mind that the geometry and material properties used in the finite element model are approximations based on either one person or an average of several people. There is a wide range of sizes and properties among individuals. The results of finite element models of biological structures should be treated as generalizations.

Similarly, modeling and stress analysis of components using the finite element method can not completely prove the adequacy of a design. Finite element analysis of a structure is merely a tool to assist in the design process, and it in no way replaces mechanical testing and analysis (in vitro and in vivo) of the device. If the results of a finite element model are to be used for component evaluation, validation of the model through comparing stress or strain values measured experimentally must be done.

■ **11.3 DESIGN CONSIDERATIONS FOR ORTHOPAEDIC IMPLANTS**

Imagine that you have just designed—in your opinion—the best elbow implant in the world! Your engineer collaborator has shown by finite element analysis that the function of an elbow with this implant in place is identical to that of a normal elbow and that the implant should last for at least 50 years, even if the patient decides to take up weight lifting as a hobby. The only problem is that your device has 15 small parts, takes a surgeon experienced in the technique about 20 hours to implant, and can be made only on a custom basis at a cost of $67,000 per implant. In addition, the manufacturer has said that the surgical jigs that must be used in implanting the device cost about $150,000 per set. So do you really have the best elbow implant in the world? The answer is, unfortunately, no. This is an extreme example, but it does point out some of the factors that one must contemplate in the design process.

11.3.1 Essence of the Design Process

Many factors must be considered simultaneously when creating a worthwhile, practical implant design. The most critical factors and a brief explanation of each are listed as follows:

1. *Appropriate function achieved.* The implant must allow the patient to achieve at least some degree of normal function. For example, a total hip replacement that does not allow a ball-and-socket type of mobility is not appropriate. However, a fusion device for the knee is very appropriate if the alternative is amputation. The appropriate degree of function required depends on the application.

2. *Stress system imposed.* If a device fails the first time the patient is fully weight bearing, the device is obviously not appropriate. A device must be designed to withstand normal loading so as not to fail in fatigue under normal circumstances. Similarly, the stresses in the contacting bone and soft tissue must be as near normal as possible. For example, a bone plate could be designed that would virtually never break, but it might cause extreme stress shielding in the bone and stick out so far that it would lead to soft tissue necrosis.

3. *Time required to function.* Implants that must function for a patient's lifetime should be designed for something like a 50-year service life if possible. Conversely, if an implant is required to function for only a limited amount of time, it will be designed differently. For example, the pins in external fixators are implanted for only a matter of weeks so that long-term fatigue may be ignored and the design may be based solely on providing adequate stiffness to keep the fracture reduced.

4. *Anatomical constraints.* The design of implants is usually severely limited by the anatomical constraints. For example, the inner diameter of the medullary canal controls the outer diameter of an intramedullary rod. If one is designing an intramedullary rod, one must consider the case of a severely overweight person with a small frame. Contraindications should be specified for such situations.

5. *Surgical convenience (ease of use).* If the technique of implantation is complicated and difficult, the chance of mistakes increases greatly. A major factor in the outcome of many implants is the technique of the orthopaedic surgeon. All implants and special jigs required for installation should be designed in such a way that the device can be implanted with minimum difficulty.

6. *Ability to manufacture on a commercial basis (manufacturability).* Many designs look impressive on paper and yield great finite element analysis results but are quite difficult for manufacturing engineers to implement. Designs must be "manufacture friendly" in order to reduce cost of production and decrease likelihood of manufacture-related defects. Many times an original design must be changed slightly to accommodate production. The impact of these changes on other considerations must be examined carefully.

7. *Simplicity.* One way to minimize the difficulties of the implantation, decrease cost, and increase manufacturability is to simplify the design as much as possible. Avoid Rube Goldberg implant designs.

8. *Removability.* Any implant can fail whether it be directly from loosening or fracture or indirectly from infection or patient sensitivity to the material. A feasible technique for removal of the implant should always be included in the design of the device.

9. *Number of parts.* As the number of parts of a device increases, so does the cost of manufacture and risk of operating-room mix-ups. The number of individual components in any implant system should be minimized.

10. *Sizes and hospital stock.* People come in many shapes and sizes, and implants must be designed in a variety of sizes to accommodate these variations. With some implants, components can be mixed and matched to produce the optimum fit for the patient. For example, in compression hip screws, different lengths of lag screws may be matched with different angles of side plate and barrel. One must take care to design foolproof components. Figure 11.3 shows an example of a poorly designed compression hip screw that was mismatched with a threaded bolt and side plate. In this example, either 1) the bolt is not long enough to go up into the threaded hole past the end of the barrel, or 2) the barrel is not long enough to encompass the full length of the threaded part of the lag screw. The lag screw is susceptible to failure at the end of the barrel because of the stress concentration at the unsupported threads in the hole.

In this age of hospital cost controls, the impact of device design on the hospital's inventory must be kept in mind. Even though it is desirable to have a well-fitted implant, hospitals may be reluctant to use a design if that design requires that a large number of different sizes be stocked. Currently, custom-sized implants are in general not economically advantageous for manufacturers or hospitals, but they may become more attractive in the future as new manufacturing techniques are developed.

11. *Material and environment.* Anything implanted in the body is subject to attack from the chemical solution of our body fluids. In addition, even though an implant may be designed well below the failure strength of the material, it may still fail due to wear. A material used in an implant design should be chosen for its biocompatibility (corrosion resistance, toxicity, tissue response, etc.), strength, stiffness, wear resistance, and fatigue and fracture properties.

12. *Cost.* In an ideal world, the cost of medical care should not be a concern. Unfortunately, we do not live in an ideal world. If a new device costs a great deal more than current devices to produce and implant, it will probably not be used unless considerable long-term cost savings can be proven. Medicare, Medicaid, and insurance companies will not reimburse the cost of surgery and an expensive implant if it is not justified monetarily in the short term. Neither the hospitals nor the vast majority of patients can afford to make up the difference between

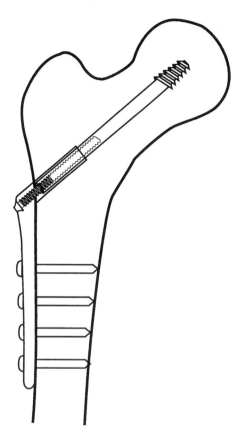

Figure 11.3. A poorly designed compression hip screw that was mismatched with a threaded bolt and side plate. The threaded hole of the lag screw that extends beyond the barrel is a potential source of premature failure.

the reimbursement and the actual cost. In order for an implant design to be practical, the cost of the device must be kept to a minimum.

■ 11.4 MECHANICS OF TOTAL HIP REPLACEMENT

Total hip replacement (THR) is considered to be a very successful surgical procedure with 5- to 10-year success rates as high as 95%. There are many mechanical considerations of THR that contribute to its success. In this section, we briefly discuss a few of the major considerations. This discussion is by no means exhaustive; the bibliography contains references that discuss these and other factors in further detail.

11.4.1 Hip Joint Forces and Moments

Chapter 2 presented a simple analysis of forces and moments about the hip. From that analysis we found that the joint reaction force on the proximal femur during the stance phase of normal gait is about three times body weight. What this simple analysis did not take into consideration is the fact that the femur is a three-dimensional structure with multidirectional forces, moments, and torques acting on it. In fact, the torques (rotational moments) about the hip can be substantial during activities such as rising from a chair or going up and down stairs. The effects of these additional loads are important to consider in the discussion of mechanical considerations of THR.

11.4.2 Type of Fixation

One of the major factors that affects the mechanics of a total hip replacement is the method of fixation used. The two categories of fixation are cemented and cementless fixation. We cannot yet make a general comparison of these two types of fixation; each type has its own limitations and strengths. Within these two categories, however, there are several subgroups with different design theories and mechanical aspects.

11.4.2.1 Cemented Fixation

Cemented fixation has been used extensively in THR since Charnley promoted the technique in the early 1960s. Newer cementing techniques have made the outcomes even more successful than the original good results. Improved techniques include porosity reduction in the cement (to increase fatigue resistance), lavage and thorough drying of the canal, pressurization through use of a cement gun, use of a medullary plug, and centralization of the stem. Failure of cemented components is thought to initiate at the stem-cement interface and to propagate by fatigue through the cement mantle. Because the cement does not chemically bond to the metal, the strength of the cement-metal interface is inherently low. Increased roughening of the stem has been promoted as a means of improving the interface strength through mechanical interlock. More discussion on the problems of bone cement as a material for fixation can be found in chapter 16, Section 16.4.

11.4.2.2 Creep in Bone Cement

An alternative approach to strengthening of the cement-metal interface in THR has been suggested in the literature. In this technique (promoted by Mr. Robin Ling), the metal implant stem should be very shiny and smooth in order to purposely reduce the mechanical interlock between the cement and the stem. In this case, the implant is set up to subside slightly in the cement through creep of the cement. This results in increased hoop stresses in the cement that are transmitted to the proximal femur. Analysis of the results of this technique are ongoing. An important mechanical consideration of this technique is that the implant must be smooth for this concept to work. A surgeon should not use a surface-roughened prosthesis in combination with the surgical procedure suggested in Mr. Ling's concepts.

11.4.2.3 Cementless Fixation

Cementless fixation through the use of biologic growth into porous surfaces or onto roughened surfaces is the alternative technique to cemented fixation. These components rely on bone (or rather, tissue) ingrowth into porous or roughened surfaces to stabilize the component. Cementless fixation is often promoted for use in younger patients because of the relatively low fatigue strength of bone cement in comparison to the imposed stresses.

One common mechanical complication of using press-fit cementless femoral components is intraoperative fracture of the femur. The need for a tight fit in the reamed canal sometimes causes hoop stresses that exceed the tensile strength of bone of the proximal femur in the circumferential direction; as a result, splitting of the bone occurs. Intraoperative fracture occurs more frequently in osteoporotic bone. Studies show that there is a significant increase in rotational instability when these fractures occur and are not stabilized with cerclage wires.

Another problem of total hip replacement (especially with cementless fixation) is stress shielding. In order to fit the femoral canal and minimize interface micromotion (which is necessary for good ingrowth), cementless components are designed with relatively large cross sections.

As discussed in chapter 6, the high rigidity of the implant reduces the stress level in the proximal femur. This may lead to bone resorption due to stress-shielding osteoporosis, which can be further aggravated by particle-induced osteolysis.

11.4.3 Positioning of the Femoral Component

The positioning of the femoral component in the femoral canal can affect the mechanics of the system. Varus or valgus placement will not only alter the mechanics of the articulation with the acetabular component but will also change the load distribution at the implant-bone interface in cementless components and cement-bone interface in cemented components.

Centralization of the stem in the canal is also important, particularly in cemented components. If the stem is not centralized, the cement mantle may be thin in one region and thick in another. The thin region is then at higher risk of fracture, and the thick region can reach higher setting temperatures than are desirable. (More on the effect of cement thickness is discussed in chapter 16, Section 16.4.)

11.4.4 Length of the Stem

There is still controversy about the appropriate length of the stem in primary uncemented components. Short stems distribute more stress to the bone while lacking the stability of the longer stem. Unique distal stem designs (such as the slotted stem) attempt to reach a compromise between these two issues.

11.4.5 Implant Material and Design Features

The current materials of choice in the United States for THR are either a cobalt-chromium (Co-Cr) alloy or a titanium (Ti) alloy for the stem, a cobalt-chromium-alloy femoral head, and a polyethylene-bearing surface. Alternative bearing surfaces such as metal-on-metal and ceramic-on-ceramic are now being explored. Polymer composite materials have also been investigated for use in THR. Each of these materials has its own mechanical advantages and disadvantages.

Titanium alloys have about half the stiffness of cobalt-chromium alloys. An implant composed of a titanium alloy would have about half the rigidity of an implant of the same size and shape but composed of a cobalt-chromium alloy. The titanium-alloy implant would therefore not shield the bone from as much of the stress as the same size and shape cobalt-chromium implant would. Whether this increased stress level in the bone is enough to substantially reduce stress-shielding-related osteoporosis is still not known. Recent studies have also suggested that the accelerated corrosion (due to the dissimilar metals; discussed in chapter 15) at the connection between a titanium stem and a cobalt-chromium head may be significant.

Composite implants have also been designed that have much lower rigidity than either titanium or cobalt-chromium femoral components. With lower rigidity, however, comes much higher micromotion at the implant-bone interface in cementless components and higher cement stresses in cemented stems. This makes bone ingrowth less likely and cement failure more probable. In addition, design of these implants to resist compressive creep failure is difficult.

Recently there has been much concern about the contribution of polyethylene wear particles to osteolysis. Attempts are being made to increase the wear resistance of polyethylene (as discussed in chapter 16). Alternative bearing surfaces have also been explored. Current metal-on-metal implants have improved metallurgy, machining, and design as compared with the original devices of the 1960s. Excellent results have been achieved with this bearing combination; however, at the present time, the economic feasibility of developing these devices for use in the United States is still not resolved.

■ 11.5 MECHANICS OF TOTAL KNEE REPLACEMENT

Total knee replacement (TKR) has also been a very successful surgical procedure. Just as with THR, there are many mechanical considerations of TKR that contribute to its success. We present and briefly discuss a few of the major points. Please refer to sources in the bibliography for a thorough review of these and other factors.

11.5.1 Knee Joint Forces and Moments

The knee is not a simple hinge. During normal gait there is motion in the anterior-posterior (A-P) and medial-lateral (M-L) directions, and rotation about the longitudinal axis (figure 11.4). All these motions and

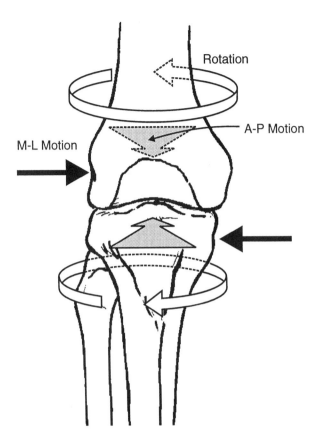

Figure 11.4. Motions of the knee joint.

the stresses generated by their constraint must be taken into account in the design of a TKR implant system. For example, in a hinged-prosthesis design, no (or very little) motion is allowed about the vertical (longitudinal) axis. Therefore, the torques responsible for this motion now act to produce shear stresses at the hinge and through the stems. This leads to excessive wear at the articulation and to failure of the stem-cement or stem-bone interfaces.

11.5.2 Design of the Tibial Component

The example of the all-polyethylene tibial component given in Section 11.1.2 shows one way in which the design of the tibial component can affect the success of the TKR. The slightly greater loading of the medial condyle must also be considered in designing the tibial component. If the prosthesis is not designed properly, a slight tilt from either the unequal loading or the misalignment of components can lead to relatively rapid failure of the polyethylene tibial tray. For example, figure 11.5a shows a flat articular surface that allows large contact areas when equal loading exists on the two condyles, but a slight tilt of the femoral component causes edge loading that reduces the area over which the load is applied. This tilt therefore results in high contact stresses (figure 11.5b). Like the flat surface design, a tibial tray that incorporates a single radius of curvature on each femoral condyle (figure 11.6a) achieves a high contact area and distributes forces well if loaded evenly. In this design, however, a slight tilt of the femoral component does not cause edge loading and still distributes the load, thus keeping contact stresses within reasonable limits (figure 11.6b).

11.5.3 Design of the Patellar Component

The patellar button is a difficult part to design. The patella is subjected to high retropatellar forces over a relatively small area. In addition, the patella is relatively thin, which places severe limitations on the thick-

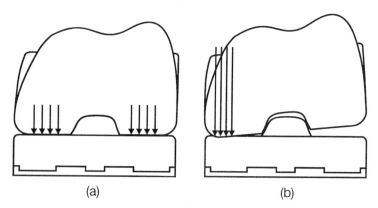

(a)   (b)

Figure 11.5. In a total knee replacement design, a flat articular surface may allow large contact areas when equal loading exists on the two condyles *(a)*. However, a slight tilt of the femoral component *(b)* causes edge loading, which results in high contact stresses. *Source:* Whiteside LA, Nagamine R, Scott W: Biomechanical Aspects of Knee Replacement Designs. In *The Knee,* vol. 2, WN Scott, Ed. Mosby, St Louis, 1994, pp. 1079–1096, 1089, figure 59.17.

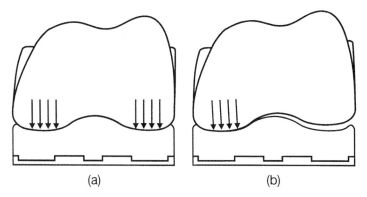

(a)   (b)

Figure 11.6. A tibial tray that incorporates a single radius of curvature on each femoral condyle *(a)* has a high contact area and distributes forces well if loaded evenly. A slight tilt of the femoral component *(b)* does not cause edge loading and keeps contact stresses within reasonable limits. *Source:* Whiteside LA, Nagamine R, Scott W: Biomechanical Aspects of Knee Replacement Designs. In *The Knee,* vol. 2, WN Scott, Ed. Mosby, St Louis, 1994, pp. 1079–1096, 1089, figure 59.18.

ness of any patellar button design. Because of these problems, wear of the polyethylene of the patellar button is still a problem. Some early metal-backed designs had polyethylene pieces that were too thin in certain regions. These regions wore rapidly and created unplanned metal-on-metal articulation that produced large quantities of metal wear particles. Recent designs are more conforming to reduce contact stresses and have thicker and more uniform polyethylene parts. Patellar component design is, however, still a challenge.

Q11: Clinical Question (Summary)

Sanza Time sustained a closed fracture of his femur that was treated by closed intramedullary rodding. Sanza did not listen to his surgeon and resumed all his vigorous normal activities almost immediately. Eleven weeks later, he showed up at the surgeon's office with a broken rod and an ununited femur fracture. How could this happen?

A11: Clinical Answer

Intramedullary rods are load-sharing devices that have tight design restraints because of the size of the medullary canal. As discussed in Section 11.1.1.1, in fracture fixation there is a race between healing of the fracture and failure of the implant. Mr. Time's intramedullary rod ran out of time before his fracture healed. This was, however, probably because of his disregard of his surgeon's instructions to avoid vigorous activity for a while. IM rods cannot be designed to withstand such forces, and it is not surprising that the device failed.

Additional Reading

Bartel DL, Bicknell VL, Wright TM: The effect of conformity, thickness and material on stresses in ultra-high molecular weight components for total joint replacement. *J Bone Joint Surg* 68A(7):1041–1051, 1986.

Beckman A: Design and Manufacturing Solutions to UHMWPE Wear in TKA. Technical Monograph 97–2010–26. Zimmer, Warsaw, Ind., 1997.

Burstein AH, Wright TM: *Fundamentals of Orthopaedic Biomechanics.* Williams & Wilkins, Baltimore, 1994.

Contact areas during flexion and rotation: Range of motion studies. Technical Monograph 6640–0–001–1. Howmedica Inc. Rutherford, N.J., 1992.

Harrigan TP, Kareh JA, O'Connor D, Burke DW, Harris WH: A finite element study of the initiation of failure of fixation in cemented femoral total hip components. *J Orthop Res* 10:134–144, 1992.

Huiskes R: Design, fixation, and stress analysis of permanent orthopaedic implants: The hip joint. In *Functional Behavior of Biomaterials, vol. II: Applications,* P. Ducheyne, G. Hastings, Eds. CRC Press, Boca Raton, Fla., pp. 121–162, 1984.

Huiskes R, Weinans H, Dalstra M: Adaptive bone remodeling and biomechanical design considerations for noncemented total hip arthroplasty. *Orthopedics* 12(9):1255–1267, 1989.

Love SF: *Planning and Creating Successful Engineered Designs.* Van Nostrand Reinhold Company, New York, 1980.

Metal on Metal Hip Prostheses: Past Performances and Future Directions. *Clin Orthop* 329S August, 1996.

Section IV: Implant Fixation. *Instruc Course Lectures* 43:233–295, 1994.

Steffenmeier SJ, Stalcup GC: UHMWPE Design Considerations in Total Hip Arthroplasty. Technical Monograph 97–2100–31. Zimmer, Inc., Warsaw, Ind., 1997.

Total Hip Replacement. NIH Consensus Statement Online, September 12–14, 1994 12(5):1–31.

Whiteside LA, Nagamine R: Biomechanical aspects of knee replacement designs. In *The Knee,* vol. 2, WN Scott, Ed. Mosby, St. Louis, pp. 1079–1096, 1994.

12

Considerations in Biomechanical Testing

CLINICAL SCENARIO: MEASURING THE STRAINS IN A FEMUR

Justin Dawn, engineering diploma in hand, was hired to work in the Orthopaedic Research Laboratory at Mega General Hospital shortly after Sanza Time was admitted with the broken femoral rod. Having seen such broken rods too many times in her long career, the chief orthopaedic surgeon at Mega General asked the staff of the research laboratory to design a stronger rod. In order to design such a device, the staff immediately recognized that some notion of the strains incurred by the current rod would have to be taken into account. Justin's first project was thus to determine what such strains might be during normal walking. How would Justin go about doing this?

Unlike other structural materials such as steel and plastic, bone is alive. When an engineer and physician team up in joint experiments, both basic mechanical testing and biological concepts must be considered in order to achieve a valid, meaningful result. This collaboration is greatly facilitated when both the engineer and physician have some knowledge of the other's specialty. In this chapter we look at some of the basic equipment and concepts used in biomechanical testing in orthopaedics.

■ 12.1 BASICS OF MECHANICAL TESTING EQUIPMENT

Several common devices are used in most biomechanical testing experiments. In this section, we cover the fundamental concepts of each device and some of the basic do's and don'ts of handling them.

12.1.1 Measurement of Strain

One of the most common tests of materials is the tensile test. In this test, a specimen of the material in question is mounted in the testing machine (figure 12.1) and pulled until it breaks. The stress and strain in

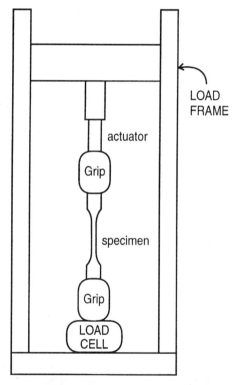

Figure 12.1. Typical testing machine setup for a tensile test. The load cell can be mounted either on the bottom (as shown) or on the top. The hydraulic actuator can move up and down under various control mechanisms to apply load to the specimen.

the material are determined and plotted to record all the important information that can be derived from this test. At first glance, one might think that measurement of the strain in the material is as simple as measuring the overall displacement of the specimen (as measured by the machine) and dividing by the original length of the specimen. Although this can give a rough estimate of strain, it is not precise enough for use in calculating elastic modulus.

Most tensile specimens are "dog-bone" shaped (figure 12.2). The wide part is gripped in the jaws of the machine and experiences com-

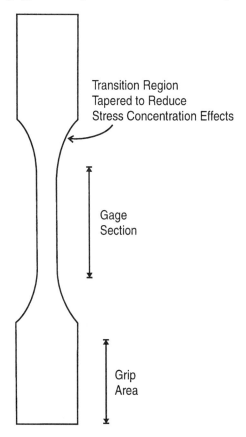

Transition Region
Tapered to Reduce
Stress Concentration Effects

Gage
Section

Grip
Area

Figure 12.2. A typical tensile specimen is tapered so that a uniform strain region is generated in the middle region (or the gage section). The appropriate size of specimens is often dictated by American Society for Testing Materials (ASTM) specifications.

plex, nonuniform stresses. Only the middle part (referred to as the gage section) has a uniform stress field; all strain measurements are made in this gage section. In principle, one could determine strain by putting marks on the gage section and measuring changes in the distance between the marks with a caliper. This is not very precise, however. Two faster and more precise measuring devices are available: the mechanical extensiometer and the electric strain gage.

12.1.1.1 Extensiometers

Extensiometers are surface-mounted mechanical devices that have two prongs or clips that attach to the specimen. The initial distance between the clips constitutes the original length, and the distance the clips move during the test is the change in length. Extensiometers are good measuring devices but can be bulky and too heavy for measuring strain in some softer materials.

12.1.1.2 Strain Gages

A more commonly used strain-measuring device is the electric *strain gage* (shown magnified in figure 12.3). Strain gages are thin wires that are parallel to each other and mounted on a thin tab of material (usually an epoxy). The strain gage is glued to the surface of the specimen at the

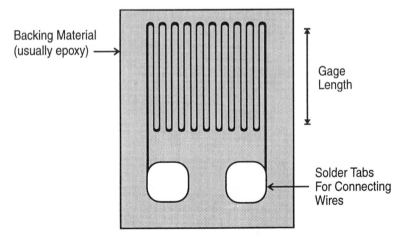

Figure 12.3. A schematic of a typical, simple strain gage is shown. Note that, in reality, there would be many more, much thinner wires than shown in this schematic.

place where strain is to be measured. The basic assumption of using the strain gage is that the strain in the strain gage is (essentially) identical to the strain on the surface of the specimen in the direction parallel to the wires. Can you think of cases (or materials) where this would not hold true?

When the strain gage is unstretched, its electrical resistance depends on the size, shape, and material of the wires. When the gage is stretched, however, the resistance increases because the wires become longer and thinner. In using the strain gage, a constant current is maintained in the wires. Under zero strain, this current requires a certain voltage:

$$\text{Voltage} = \text{current} \times \text{resistance or } V = I \times R$$

When the gage wires are stretched, the resistance increases an amount ΔR, so the voltage must be increased by an amount ΔV to maintain a constant current:

$$\Delta V = I \times \Delta R$$

The change in voltage can be measured and correlated to the amount of strain in the wires. Through the magic of signal conditioning, special strain gage equipment, and calibration numbers supplied by the manufacturers, one can correlate the change in voltage across the strain gage to the strain quite precisely. Strain gage data are usually acquired in units of microstrain, or strain times 10^6. Reading strain in microstrain units yields results that are easier to read, interpret, and report. For example, the maximum strain in the femoral component of a hip prosthesis might be 0.00127. This corresponds to 1,270 microstrain units, or 1,270 $\mu\varepsilon$.

Several assumptions are made in using strain gages. As already mentioned, we assume that the strain in the gage is the same as the strain on the surface of the specimen. This is a poor assumption for very soft materials (such as soft tissues) in which the gage may actually significantly reinforce the material.

The strain gage must also be very well bonded to the specimen. If the attachment is not good, the gage will not reflect the true surface strain. For example, if the glue softens (as it may in elevated temperatures or in solution), the strain in the gage will be less than in the actual specimen.

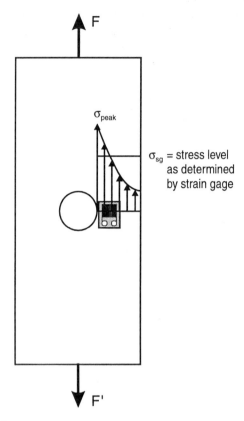

Figure 12.4. As shown in this diagram, data from a strain gage placed next to a hole (or other stress-raising defect) will not reflect the high strain at the edge of the hole. The strain measured will be an average of the entire area of the strain gage wires.

One must always be aware that the strain gage averages the strain measurement over the area of the wires in the gage. Figure 12.4 illustrates one of the problems that this averaging can generate. If the local strains vary sharply, that is, have a very steep gradient, the strain gage will not provide an accurate view of the strain distribution. This is the case shown in figure 12.4, where a hole in a bone plate will cause stress concentration (see chapter 8). The strain gage would only average the strain and would not be able to measure the peak strain at the very edge of the hole. Such strain averaging is not a problem when the strain distribution is relatively uniform.

What if one does not know the direction in which the important strain lies? Placing one strain gage on the specimen will then give the strain only in the direction of the gage, which may not be the actual maximum strain at that site. When the direction of the maximum strain is unknown, a special strain gage called a rosette is used. The typical rosette consists of three strain gages that are either stacked on top of each other or grouped tightly together in specified angular orientations. The strain readings from these three gages can be analyzed to yield the magnitude and direction of the maximum strain at the location of the gages.

12.1.1.3 Other Strain-Measuring Devices

Although strain gages are wonderful tools, they have some limitations. Suppose one wants to measure the strain distribution in a complex structure such as the pelvis. Hundreds of strain gages would be required to map the complex strain pattern in these bones. Another limitation is the time and skill required to mount strain gages. Proper gluing of strain gages onto the specimen surface and wiring into the signal-conditioning equipment is an acquired skill and is neither easy nor quick. The idea of installing a hundred strain gages on a pelvis is enough to make even the best technician consider quitting! In these cases, alternative full-field methods of strain measurement may be of benefit.

The two most important techniques of full-field strain measurement are surface photoelasticity and thermoelastic stress analysis (TSA). Photoelasticity depends on the property of birefringence exhibited by certain polymers. If polarized light is passed through a birefringent material and the material is then subjected to strain, both light and dark bands appear. These bands are called fringes, and the local strains can be determined from the fringe pattern. To reveal the strain patterns in a complex object like the pelvis, the object must first be painted with a reflective metallic coating, which in turn is covered with a film of the birefringent polymer. The structure is then viewed under polarized light that passes through the birefringent film, reflects off the metallic coating, and passes back through the film again. When a load is applied to the structure, the strains produced in the film give rise to fringes that are photographed and analyzed. This technique requires that the coatings be well bonded so that the strains in the film are the same as the strains in the surface of the structure beneath. This technique is most useful for identifying the position and approximate magnitudes of the highest strains in complex structures.

Thermoelastic stress analysis utilizes the thermoelastic effect in materials. A specimen is cyclically loaded, and an infrared camera measures minute temperature changes in a material. These temperature changes correlate to strain changes in the structure. Just as with strain gages, each of these techniques has its advantages and limitations.

The details of using these tests are not be discussed in this text. These techniques are mentioned as examples so that you will know that there are many alternatives and unique methods for determining the state of stress and strain in structures.

12.1.2 Measurement of Displacement

Many different transducers are available to measure displacements. These transducers can be separated into contacting and noncontacting categories. The most common contacting displacement-measuring devices are variable differential transformers that consist of an electric circuit, including a coil and a magnetic core that is moved inside the coil. The impedance of the circuit provides an output voltage that is proportional to the position of the core. Variable differential transformers can be either linear (LVDT) or rotational (RVDT). These devices come with a variety of signal-conditioning methods, shapes, and accuracies and can usually be used with standard data-acquisition equipment, after some calibration. Noncontacting displacement-measuring devices usually use magnetic fields to sense an object's changes in position.

12.1.3 Measuring Force: The Load Cell

The load cell is the most common device used to measure force. The load cell consists of a structural element—a bar or beam with strain gages attached. When a load is applied to the cell, the element experiences strains that are sensed by the gages. It is then a simple matter to apply known loads (e.g., weights) to the cell and calibrate the strain gage output voltage in units of force. Thus force is measured indirectly by measuring the strain in the element. Figure 12.5 shows a simple representation of how this indirect calculation of force might work.

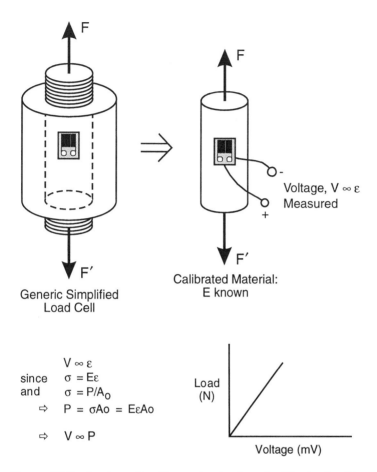

Figure 12.5. A schematic of how a load cell works. The load cell has a piece of calibrated material with a strain gage on it. Force is measured by relating the voltage of the strain gage to load.

Load cells are designed to measure force in a specific manner. For example, some load cells measure only compression force. Others can measure uniaxial forces in either tension or compression. Biaxial load cells are usually designed to measure an axial force and a moment, such as torque. One very important concept to remember when using a load cell is that it should never be subjected to any mode of loading other than that for which it was designed. For example, if one has a uniaxial tension-compression load cell, one should never subject it to bending when performing an experiment. Doing so will not only risk damaging it permanently, but will result in erroneous readings of the axial force.

Load cells are also designed to withstand a given load level. The cost of the load cell depends in part on its accuracy and ability to measure biaxial forces; these transducers can range in price from $50 to more than $15,000. If the load or moment applied to a load cell exceeds its design maximum, the beams inside the cell may undergo plastic deformation and be permanently deformed. If this happens, the voltages output by the load cell are no longer in calibration, and the load cell is sometimes irreparably damaged. A compromised load cell cannot be trusted to yield accurate information. Damaging a load cell can be very costly in terms of ruining the device, collecting bad data, wasting valuable specimens and time, and, worst of all, creating the potential for reporting erroneous data.

12.1.4 Measuring Pressure

Pressure can be thought of as the stress generated over a surface by a distributed force. Typical examples are the pressure between the skin of a patient's buttocks and the surface of a wheelchair cushion and also the pressure between the skin of an amputee's stump and the inside of the amputee's prosthesis socket. A common technique for measuring pressure between two contacting surfaces is the use of pressure-sensitive film. Just as with load cells, different films are designed to measure varying pressure levels. We present only a simple explanation of how this method works.

Pressure-sensitive film consists of plastic sheets with "ink-filled" capsules between them. The sheets are placed between contacting surfaces where pressure is to be measured (for example, between the radius and scaphoid in a cadaver), and load is applied across the joint. The "ink capsules" are of multiple sizes that are designed to burst at given pressure levels. If the film is exposed to a low pressure (within its specified range), only the low-pressure capsules will burst, and the stain intensity will be light. If a high pressure is applied, many capsules will burst, and the stain will be heavy. The intensity of the stain can be calibrated within ranges, and the distribution of pressures over the test film can be determined. Only pressure ranges are determined in this method. Although simple in concept, pressure-sensitive film can be very challenging to calibrate and interpret with confidence.

■ 12.2 CONSIDERATIONS IN TESTING SYNTHETIC BIOMATERIALS

Special considerations apply when synthetic biomaterials are tested. For example, implanted biomaterials are used at body temperature. Will the material one is testing behave the same at room temperature as it does at body temperature? If proper thought is not given to testing conditions in advance of the experiment, it is possible to complete an entire test series that results in material data that are not representative of the conditions of interest. In this section, some basic ideas about testing conditions are presented. These ideas are by no means exhaustive but are given as "food for thought" to be considered in designing one's own testing protocol.

12.2.1 Testing Temperature and Environment

The temperature and environment of a mechanical test can have a substantial effect on the results obtained. For this reason it would be ideal to test all implant materials and devices at 37°C, that is, body temperature, in simulated body fluids. Unfortunately, this can be an expensive proposition. Simulated body fluids can mean anything from a simple isotonic saline solution to whole blood. Moreover, a chamber must be built to contain the solution in contact with the specimen, and a heater and temperature controller must be provided to maintain the environment at the desired temperature. In addition to the cost of building and maintaining these chambers, one must recognize that the chambers interfere with specimen mounting and present an ever present threat of leakage, which can severely damage expensive electrical and mechanical equipment. Obviously one does not get involved in such testing unless it is absolutely necessary. The question then arises, when is it necessary? How does one know when it is important to go to the expense of environmentally correct testing and when can one do faster and easier testing?

As a rule of thumb, the properties of metals are not significantly affected by the difference between the temperature of the body environment and room temperature. Static and most dynamic tests of metallic biomaterials can be conducted at room temperature in air. If corrosion or friction is of concern, then bioanalogue fluids must be used. Isotonic saline solution may be suitable if the effect of corrosion on mechanical properties is being investigated (for example, corrosion fatigue), but a synovial-fluid analogue such as blood plasma may be required if metal-on-metal wear in a prosthetic joint is being studied.

The testing of polymeric materials must be approached with more caution. Polymers are much more sensitive to small temperature changes than are metals and are much more likely to interact with the environment. For example, polymers whose glass transition temperature is near 37°C may have markedly different mechanical properties at room temperature than at body temperature. Other polymers may—on exposure to the biological environment—absorb water molecules that soften or plasticize the material. Thus a polymer component that has been implanted for even a few days may be measurably weaker than its nonexposed duplicate. In general the static properties of polymers may be determined in air at room temperature for purposes of preliminary screening and comparison and to assess batch-to-batch variability. Tests in which time-dependent properties (for example, fatigue or creep) are being measured, and tests of actual implants should always be conducted at 37°C in a suitable bioanalogue fluid. The debate on what solution is appropriate for use in testing has not yet been completely resolved. In addition to water molecules, some constituents of body fluids (proteins, lipids, etc.) may be absorbed by a polymer and change their mechanical behavior. In most cases, either isotonic saline or diluted serum are used. For this reason, it is *very* important to report all test conditions in detail.

> ➤ Time-dependent mechanical properties of polymers are sensitive to testing temperature and environment.

12.2.2 Testing Rate and Frequency

In most situations, the properties of metals are not dependent on the rate of testing. In static testing, the strain rate or load rate does not materially effect the results unless very high-rate impact loading is involved. Likewise, fatigue testing of implant metals can be conducted at elevated frequencies, except when corrosion-accelerated fatigue testing is performed.

Conversely, testing rate is very important for biopolymers. All static testing should be performed at a stroke, strain, or load rate similar to that which is experienced by the part in vivo. Furthermore, all time-dependent tests (such as fatigue tests) should be done at frequencies similar to those experienced in the body under normal loading conditions. In general, frequencies of 1–2 Hz (one hertz equals one cycle per second) are used to test biopolymers. More rapid testing leads to specimen warming, which decreases strength and causes significant changes in fatigue life. Low frequencies create logistical difficulties, however. To conduct endurance-limit or wear-rate tests to 10^7 cycles, a test running at 1 Hz would take about 111 days! Dynamic testing of human-made polymers can be wearing on one's patience as well as on the specimen!

> ➢ Mechanical properties of polymers are sensitive to rate of testing.

12.2.3 Aging and Heat Treatment of Materials

Once again, metals do not change with time except when corrosion is involved. A metal part can sit on the hospital shelf for many years, and no change in fatigue life will occur. The high-temperature heat treatments used in the fabrication of metal implants do, however, change their mechanical behavior. Metal specimens intended to represent an implant should always receive the same heat treatment as the implant received during fabrication.

Plastics are, however, sensitive to aging. For example, the properties of bone cement change during the first 24 hours after mixing because polymerization (or curing) of the polymer is still taking place. Ultra-high molecular weight polyethylene material (UHMWPE) can also undergo changes in material properties with time (see chapter 16), particularly if it has been sterilized by gamma irradiation. In general, specimens of biopolymers should always be tested under the aging and heat-treatment conditions used in manufacture.

12.2.4 ASTM Specifications (or Standards) for Testing Biomaterials

A set of recommendations for standardized testing of materials is provided by the American Society for Testing and Materials (ASTM) for many tests and materials. These specifications recommend specimen shapes, testing rates, environments, and so on so that all investigators can conduct comparable tests. There is a special ASTM committee (F4) that specifies testing methods specifically for biomaterials and implant devices. Whenever possible, these specifications should be followed so that one's data can be compared with previous work. The ASTM specifications can be found in any engineering library.

■ 12.3 CONSIDERATIONS IN TESTING BIOLOGICAL MATERIALS

In general, biological materials are sensitive to rate of testing, frequency, temperature, environmental solution, and storage time. The testing conditions and the way the specimen is handled are very important when studying biological materials such as bone, soft tissues, and cartilage. This section is not intended to be a definitive guide on testing biological materials; entire books are dedicated to that subject. Here we merely point out general guidelines for testing and leave the "meat" of the subject for the reader to find in other sources.

> ➢ Biological materials are sensitive to rate of testing, temperature, environment, and age.

12.3.1 Proper Freezer Storage and Handling

Use of fresh frozen tissue makes testing of biological materials feasible. If completely fresh, unfrozen specimens were required for valid testing, chances are that much less work would be accomplished in this field. Freezing of tissues must, however, be done with care. Specimens must be wrapped in towels soaked with saline solution and sealed in a watertight pouch to keep them hydrated; bone and other tissues will get "freezer burned" just like hamburger that is not properly wrapped. Even tissues that are properly wrapped will change with regard to mechanical properties if stored in a freezer for a long period of time. Some sources recommend storing biological specimens no longer than 6 weeks in a normal freezer before testing. While it is out of the freezer and thawed, the tissue must be kept wet with saline solution at all times. Specimen testing should also be completed within 6 hours after thawing to prevent significant changes in mechanical properties caused by tissue degradation.

12.3.2 Hydrodynamic Effects

In our body, all our tissues are surrounded by fluids. In fact, a large percentage of the composition of our tissues is water and other fluids. When a piece of tissue is excised from an organ, it is no longer subjected to the same hydrodynamic effects (that is, effects from flow and pressurization of the fluids) as it was in the body. Hydrodynamic effects are, however, difficult to reproduce in testing.

■ 12.4 CONSIDERATIONS IN TESTING ORTHOPAEDIC DEVICES

One golden rule applies in the testing of orthopaedic devices: If it is not that way in the body, it is not appropriate for the test. In other words, the test must mimic the mechanical loading experienced by the device in vivo, or the test is meaningless. For example, why would one ever do pure tensile testing of a compression hip screw when one knows that the primary mode of loading on the device in vivo is bending? Such a test may be easy to do, but the results are completely useless. Some ASTM specifications exist for testing orthopaedic devices such as bone plates and hip implants; however, the vast majority of implants have no recommended, standard test protocol. Tests of orthopaedic devices devised by the investigator should be modeled as closely as possible on the conditions in the body. When ASTM specifications are not available, one should first review the literature to see what other investigators have used for mechanical testing protocols for the orthopaedic device in question. Much can be learned from the experiences and difficulties of previous investigators. If a test protocol for a specific device is well established in the literature (even though no formal ASTM specification is available), it is a good idea to use that protocol unless there is an obvious mistake in the testing setup. In this way, one may be able to compare one's results with those in the literature.

If no previous studies (or only limited ones) have been done or if one is dissatisfied with the existing protocols, then one must justify one's own protocol through comparison with in vivo conditions. For example, in the clinical scenario at the beginning of this chapter, after doing a thorough literature review, Justin might want to implant one of the current intramedullary (IM) nails in a fresh frozen cadaver femur. He should consider loading it according to the testing protocol developed by Harris and Oh (1978) for loads across the femur in one-legged stance. However, before implanting the rod, Justin should mount rosette strain gages along the rod at the fracture site in order to determine the strains that exist in the rod under these loading conditions. From this he could obtain a good idea of the maximum strains that occur in the current rod, and he could use this knowledge to help determine how much stiffer (i.e., thicker) the new rod should be to achieve the improved performance desired by the chief orthopaedic surgeon.

Q12: Clinical Question (Summary)

Justin Dawn needed to determine the strains on a femoral rod during walking. How would he go about doing this?

A12: Clinical Answer

A brief answer to this question can be found in Section 12.4, Considerations in Testing Orthopaedic Devices. Justin should utilize both existing test protocols and modifications to the protocol to determine the strains on the IM nail.

Additional Reading

Ducheyne P, Hastings G (Eds): *Functional Behavior of Biomaterials, Vol. I: Fundamentals.* CRC Press, Boca Raton, Fla.,1984.

Effects of Cast Vitallium Alloy and Prosthesis Design on Femoral Component Strength. Technical Monograph 6270–0-008. Howmedica Inc., Rutherford, N.J., 1993.

Jennings J, Stalcup G: Fatigue Test Comparison of Spiked Acetabular Implants. Technical Monograph 97–6200–07. Zimmer, Warsaw, Ind., 1997.

Oh I, Harris WH: Proximal strain distribution in the loaded femur. *J Bone Joint Surg* 60A(1):75–85, 1978.

von Recum AF (Ed): *Handbook of Biomaterials Evaluation: Scientific, Technical, and Clinical Testing of Implant Materials.* Macmillan, New York, 1986.

13

Biomaterials Basics

CLINICAL SCENARIO: FRACTURE OF A CERAMIC FEMORAL HEAD

Dr. J. P. Curmudgeon, chief of orthopaedic surgery at Mega General Hospital had done thousands of total hip arthroplasty operations with generally excellent results. Still, he was constantly in search of new and better methods of dealing with the problems of the arthritic hip. When he learned about the frequent use in Japan of a ceramic femoral head replacement, he contacted a Japanese colleague in Tokyo and went there to learn the technique. His gracious host invited him to assist in the operating room and even handed him the ceramic femoral head when it was time to insert it into the patient. Unfortunately, Dr. Curmudgeon did not realize how slippery the device was and dropped it onto the operating room floor, where it shattered. Needless to say, Dr. Curmudgeon was highly embarrassed. Was the ceramic head defective? If not, could something so brittle be expected to function as a hip replacement?

In the first 12 chapters of this book, our purpose was to understand the principals of mechanics as they apply to orthopaedics. We paid special attention to the mechanical functioning of devices and structures (including the musculoskeletal system), but we spent little time on the materials from which these systems are constructed. The structure, properties, and response to service conditions of the materials used are as important to the performance of a device as are its mechanics. For this reason, the final chapters of this book are devoted to an examination of the structure and properties of the principal materials encountered in orthopaedics. Some of the basic characteristics of solids—particularly the nature of their interatomic bonding—will be reviewed in this chapter as an introduction to the subsequent chapters that deal with specific materials.

■ 13.1 DEFINITION OF THE SOLID STATE AND THE NATURE OF INTERATOMIC BONDS

In nature, carbon occurs in two solid forms: diamond and graphite. These two forms differ in their interatomic bonding and in the way their atoms are arranged, that is, in their crystal structure. As a result of these structural differences, they have markedly different properties. Diamond is colorless and transparent, whereas graphite is black and opaque; diamond is an electrical insulator, whereas graphite is a good conductor. The hardest of all materials, diamond is used as an abrasive for grinding and cutting, but graphite is soft enough to be used as a lubricant. Because atomic and molecular structure has such an obvious and profound influence on the properties of materials, metallurgists and solid-state physicists are preoccupied with structure-property relationships. The following discussion explains how the properties of materials depend on their atomic and molecular structure.

In considering the vast array of substances in nature, it is helpful to begin by dividing all materials into their three naturally occurring states of aggregation: solid, liquid, and gas.

13.1.1 Gases

At temperatures above absolute zero, the atoms or molecules of a gas speed through space with a velocity that increases with temperature. When such atoms collide with each other or with the walls of a container, they almost always rebond elastically and keep on going. There is essentially no attraction between the atoms or molecules of a gas. Their thermally induced kinetic energy (the energy associated with a moving mass) is sufficient to keep them always on the move. For this reason, gases expand to fill their containers uniformly, and their elastic collisions with the walls of the containers are the source of the pressure that inflates balloons and powers the pistons of gasoline engines.

13.1.2 Liquids

In a liquid, there is a mild to strong attraction between atoms or molecules, with the result that, over time, each one is surrounded by an average of 11 or 12 neighbors that all touch each other; that is, they are near neighbors. Their thermal excitation at room temperature is still significant, however, and causes them to vibrate in place and to migrate past each other (though much more slowly than the passage of atoms in a gas). Because of the interatomic attraction, the atoms of a liquid do not have sufficient kinetic energy to expand and fill the whole volume of a container but are condensed in the bottom of the vessel, where they can maintain a large number of near neighbors. The interatomic bonding is not sufficient to resist the force of gravity, however, and liquids slump until they have a smooth, flat surface perpendicular to the gravity-force vector.

Liquids are much denser than gases because of the close packing (touching) of the near neighbors; in fact, they are very nearly as dense as solids and, like solids, have unique densities at a given temperature. Nonetheless, the arrangement of near neighbors is not geometrically perfect, so the orderly arrangement of the atoms does not persist over long distances (i.e., 4 or 5 atomic diameters). Liquids are the least well understood of the three states of matter.

13.1.3 Solids

Because the atoms of solids exert stronger forces of attraction on each other than do the atoms of liquids, they become organized into very nearly perfect three-dimensional arrangements that persist over very long distances (e.g., thousands of atomic diameters). When the atoms of a substance are arranged in an orderly pattern that repeats in three dimensions, the aggregate is called a crystal. Most of the substances commonly recognized as solids are crystalline; these include all metals and very nearly all ceramics and minerals. In some cases, the individual crystals are so large that they can be recognized by the unaided eye (for example, salt crystals and diamonds). More rarely, metal crystals can be seen directly. The crazy-quilt patterns sometimes seem on the surface of galvanized (zinc-coated) sheet metal are, in fact, made up of large flat crystals of zinc. Usually, however, the constituent crystals of metals and ceramics are of microscopic dimensions (0.1 μm to perhaps

100 μm), so they cannot be seen with the unaided eye; for this reason, the crystalline nature of solids often goes unappreciated.

In addition to establishing the long-range order of crystallinity, the strong bonds of the solid state make these materials very resistant to deformation when external forces are applied. Not only do crystalline solids not slump under the influence of gravity, but much greater forces generally produce only minute distortions, and even these vanish as soon as the applied force is removed. This is the elastic behavior we have discussed previously.

■ 13.2 MAGNITUDES OF BOND STRENGTHS

To avoid confusion later, we should note at this point that both solid bonds and liquid bonds occur with a range of strengths. The bonding between carbon atoms in diamond or between aluminum and oxygen in aluminum oxide (Al_2O_3; e.g., sapphire) is very much greater than that between sodium (Na) and chlorine (Cl) in rock salt, or between aluminum atoms in metallic aluminum. Macroscopically, we recognize these differences in bond strengths as differences in either bulk strength or hardness. Diamond will scratch steel (mostly iron atoms), steel will scratch aluminum, and aluminum will scratch the mineral talc.

For liquids, we commonly recognize differences in interatomic bond strengths by how fast the liquid will slump under the influence of gravity at around room temperature. For many liquids (e.g., water, alcohol, and mercury), this slumping is almost instantaneous. For some, such as oils and syrups, slumping can be recognized as a process that requires a finite, albeit a short, time period. For still other liquids, such as grease, wax, and tar (on a hot day), complete slumping may require many hours or even days. In the extreme, there is a family of liquid substances with such strong internal bonding that noticeable slumping may take decades or centuries. These are called amorphous solids, and glass is an example. For all practical purposes, these substances are solids because they hold their shape under the influence of gravity and even much larger forces for longer than anyone would care to watch. (The window panes of medieval cathedrals are measurably thicker at the bottom than at the top due to slumping, but that process took 400–700 years!) Many glasses, especially those based on silicon oxide, are stronger than the softer metals (such as aluminum and copper) and will even scratch steel. Thus, the strongest liquid bonds are comparable to the weaker (crystalline) solid bonds. Despite this robust strength, however, glasses do not possess long-range internal structure; because they are not crystalline, they are called amorphous solids. Furthermore, their slumping behavior differs from that of ordinary liquids only in the rate at which it proceeds.

■ 13.3 CHANGES IN STATE

Most substances can change from one state to another (e.g., solids melt and liquids boil). If the environment is changed in a direction that promotes less dense atomic packing (such as raising the temperature or lowering the pressure), solids tend to melt and liquids tend to boil. How do liquids boil? As heat (energy) is added to a liquid, its atoms or molecules vibrate more rapidly. Increasing the rate of vibration is equivalent to increasing the kinetic energy of the atoms, which is sensed as an increase in temperature. The average velocity associated with these vibrations also increases. If the kinetic energy is increased enough, the atomic velocity is eventually sufficient to overcome the attraction of neighboring atoms (i.e., break the interatomic bonds), and atoms escape through the surface of the liquid and enter the gaseous phase. There is a precise energy at which this will happen (i.e., where the vibrational velocity is just great enough for the atoms to escape). This energy is a measure of the bond strength; for high bond strengths, much energy must be supplied, and the liquid boils at a high temperature. By analogy, strong solids have high melting points.

From this discussion, one can easily see why bond strengths are usually discussed in terms of energy (i.e., the energy required to rupture the bond). The characteristics of the three states of matter, including glass, are summarized in table 13.1.

■ 13.4 TYPES OF SOLID BONDS

The bonds responsible for the cohesion of solids arise from interactions between the valence electrons of the constituent atoms. There are three types of strong or primary bonds: ionic, covalent, and metallic.

Table 13.1 Characteristics of gases, liquids, solids and glasses at room temperature and pressure

State	Bond strength	Structure	Density	Conformation	Examples
Gas	Very weak (elastic collisions dominate)	None	Generally low; depends only on the number of atoms or molecules in a given container	Expands to fill the volume of the vessel in which it is contained	Air Helium Methane
Liquid	Medium to strong	Short range (near neighbor touching) only	Generally high; controlled by short-range order, does not depend on volume of container	Fills container to a uniform level	Water Alcohol Mercury
Solid	Strong to very strong	Long range nearly perfect order in 3-D (crystalline)	Generally slightly greater than that of similar liquids	Does not conform to the shape of its container, resists gravity and much stronger forces	Aluminum oxide Titanium Stainless steel Co-Cr alloy
Amorphous solid	Strong	Short range only (not crystalline)	Generally a little less than other solids	Rate of container filling too slow to be of practical importance	Glass

13.4.1 Ionic Bonding

Most of the periodic table of the elements can be divided into substances that are either electron donors or electron acceptors. Electron donors have one, two, three, or, in some cases, four loosely bound electrons in their outermost valence shells, which they readily give up in chemical reactions. These materials are metals. Electron-acceptor elements have five, six, or seven valence electrons, so their valence shells are nearly full, that is, they are approaching the stable octet configuration. It is energetically favorable for these elements to accept electrons, and as such they are nonmetals.

An ionic bond is formed when an electron-donor atom transfers one or more of its valence electrons to an electron-acceptor atom. The donor (metal) atom thus becomes a cation, and the acceptor (nonmetal) atom becomes an anion. These oppositely charged ions then attract each other strongly and establish the ionic bond that holds them together and substantially reduces the energy of the pair. Ionic solids, of course, are composed of many anions and cations, which are arranged so as to minimize the overall energy of the assemblage. To achieve this, each cation is surrounded by many anions as possible, and each anion is surrounded by as many cations as possible. An ionic bond exists between each contacting cation-anion pair. This arrangement is very regular and orderly and repeats indefinitely in all directions, with the result that the whole collection constitutes a crystal (figure 13.1). Furthermore, the total number of positive charges associated with the cations is just equal to the total number of negative charges associated with the anions; overall, therefore, the crystal is electrically neutral, as one would expect. The crystal structure depicted in figure 13.1 is that of sodium chloride; each ion is surrounded by six nearest neighbors of opposite charge. This crystal structure has cubic symmetry, which is common to a great many ionic solids. Other arrangements are possible, however. For example, both aluminum oxide and hydroxyapatite (the mineral phase of bone and teeth) are ionic crystals with complex hexagonal crystal structures.

In ionic crystals, the electrons that were loosely bound in the original donor (metal) atoms are now tightly held by the anions and are, therefore, unavailable to act as charge carriers. For this reason, ionic solids are poor conductors of electricity. Sodium chloride (NaCl) is an example of an ionic solid with relatively weak bonding. During dissolution in water, the polar water molecule easily disrupts the bonds between the Na^+ and the Cl^- ions. Aluminum oxide, on the other hand, is

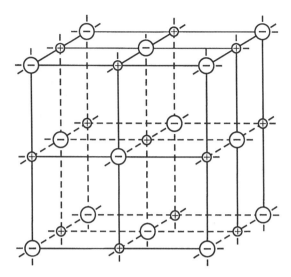

Figure 13.1. Model of sodium chloride (NaCl) crystal structure. This is an exploded model where the distances between ions is large compared to the ions themselves. This is done so that the three-dimensional nature of the structure can be easily seen. The locations of the ionic bonds are shown as lines (solid or dashed). The actual crystal extends indefinitely (that is, for thousands of ions) in every direction, with the cations and anions alternating along each bond direction. Furthermore, the ions are in reality so large that they touch their nearest neighbors at each bond location. Each cation (sodium), is surrounded by six anions (chlorine). If the crystal model alone is allowed to grow by the addition of more cations and anions, it will become obvious that each anion will also be surrounded by six ions of opposite charge, that is, cations.

an ionic solid that is not only completely resistant to dissolution in water but has such strong bonding that it is one of the hardest, highest-melting-point materials known. These strong bonds played an important and paradoxical role in the accidental fracture of Dr. Curmudgeon's ceramic femoral head, which was, in fact, made of aluminum oxide.

13.4.2 Covalent Bonding

Although most elements are either metals or nonmetals, there is one important and interesting element with a valence of four that falls at the

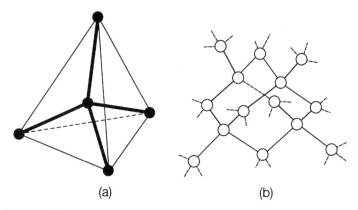

(a)   (b)

Figure 13.2. *(a)* Model of tetrahedral double bonds arranged around a central atom. *(b)* Model of diamond crystal structure in which each atom has four of its nearest neighbors arranged in tetrahedra.

boundary between these two classes. This element is carbon, and its atoms are neither electron donors nor acceptors; rather, they share pairs of valence electrons to form covalent bonds. Because each atom has four valence electrons, it can establish covalent bonds with four nearest neighbors. Close packing of these neighbors about a central atom leads to a tetrahedral arrangement (figure 13.2a). When these tetrahedra are repeated indefinitely in three dimensions, a crystal of carbon (diamond) is formed (figure 13.2b). Again the valence electrons are tightly held, this time in the vicinity of the covalent bonds.

In diamond, these electrons are so tightly held that they are not available to act as charge carriers; thus, diamond is an electrical insulator. These strong bonds are also responsible for the great strength of diamond.

13.4.3 Metallic Bonding

The third class of strong interatomic bonding occurs in metal crystals. Because the atoms involved in this kind of bonding are all electron donors, neither sharing nor transferring of electrons is involved. Rather, the valence electrons are more or less free to circulate about the donor atoms—or, more accurately, ions—which are fixed at their crystal-lattice sites. Bonding arises from the attraction between the positively charged ions and the electrons, which, on a time-average basis, are evenly distributed between them. At first, this model might not seem quite as intuitively satisfying as the models of ionic and covalent bonding. Nonetheless, this construct—called the electron-gas or free-electron model—has successfully explained many of the physical properties of metals. The free electrons are responsible for both the high electrical and thermal conductivity of metals and also their high chemical reactivity.

Another important property of metals is their ductility. When an external stress is applied to a metal crystal, some of its ions are displaced to new lattice sites (i.e., strain occurs without complete disruption of the bonds involved). This is possible because the electrons are free to accommodate these changes and can maintain the strength of the bonds as the displacements occur. The localized electrons in ionic and covalent bonds are not free to make such adjustments, and these materials do not exhibit true ductile behavior. Furthermore, during plastic deformation, the displaced ions take up new lattice sites, and the induced strain persists even when the applied stress is removed. This behavior contrasts with elastic strain, which is recovered when the applied stress is removed.

13.4.4 Weak Bonding

Many polymeric materials are composed of long, chainlike organic molecules in which the basic molecular units, or mers, are bound by strong covalent bonds. If there are no covalent cross-links between these chains, then the strength of the bulk polymer depends on the weak van der Waals or hydrogen bonds that operate between the chains. These weak bonds have less than 10% of the strength of the covalent bonds within the chains, and such polymers are markedly weaker than most other solids.

■ 13.5 MATERIALS OF CONSTRUCTION

The three primary bond types correspond roughly to three classes of construction materials: ceramics, metals, and polymers. Two of these—metals and polymers (see chapters 14 and 16, respectively)—have been widely exploited in the fabrication of implants, devices, and instruments for orthopaedics. Ceramics, on the other hand, have not fared as well.

13.5.1 Ceramics

Typical ceramics are hard, brittle, inert materials, usually metal oxides, that exhibit predominantly ionic bonding. Because these materials are produced by chemical reaction, they are already in a low-energy state, and their potential for further reaction is minimal. For this reason, they are by far the most chemically inert of materials, and, accordingly, their most compelling attribute as potential implants is their unparalleled biocompatibility. Lured on by the promise of biological acceptance, numerous attempts have been made to adapt a variety of ceramics for use as implants. After some 30 years of effort, however, none of these materials has achieved a secure place in the orthopaedic armamentarium. Why should this be? The answer, in a word, is *brittleness.* All commercially produced materials contain defects of various kinds, including microscopic pores, cracks, foreign particles, and chemical inhomogeneities. When a stress is applied, these defects locally enhance stress and eventually cause cracks to form. In metals, plastic deformation occurs under the influence of these locally intense stresses, and the cracks are blunted at least temporarily. Only when macroscopic plastic deformation has progressed to a more or less advanced state do these cracks start to grow and contribute to complete fracture in metal components. In ceramics, the ionic bonds do not permit the local rearrangement of ions necessary for plastic deformation to proceed. As a result, inherent defects are not blunted when stress is applied, and the strength of a ceramic part depends on the size and distribution of defects, not on the strength of its primary bonds. Because the size distribution and orientation of defects is probabilistic in nature, the design strength of ceramics parts must be expressed in statistical terms. In fact, a completely new field of structural design called fracture mechanics has been developed to do just this. Unfortunately, it has never been possible to fabricate cost-effective ceramic implants with low enough failure probabilities to satisfy the high-stress demands of orthopaedics. No doubt, an unusually large defect was present in the ball Dr. Curmudgeon dropped, and the stresses developed on striking the floor were great enough to trigger catastrophic growth of this crack. Perhaps Dr. Curmudgeon inadvertently did the patient a favor.

Before closing this chapter on ceramics, we should say a few words about two ceramic materials that may yet prove to have futures in orthopaedics: carbon and hydroxyapatite.

13.5.1.1 Carbon

As indicated earlier, carbon is an element that exhibits extraordinarily strong covalent bonds. Because it is an element and not a compound, it is not technically a ceramic; however, it is usually grouped with the ceramics because of its great hardness, brittleness, and inertness, especially as an implant material. The persistent interest in carbon arises from the fact that it can be produced in the form of relatively cheap fibers. The carbon atoms in these fibers do not take up the tetrahedral structure of diamond but rather have a complex arrangement related to the hexagonal structure of graphite. Nonetheless, these fibers are extraordinarily strong and stiff. It is possible to capitalize on these exceptional mechanical properties by incorporating the fibers into polymer matrix composites that exhibit very useful properties at reasonable cost. In particular, it may be possible to fabricate hip endoprostheses from carbon-fiber-reinforced composites of a stiffness similar to bone. This would be a desirable advance because the adverse remodeling of the proximal femur that often occurs in total hip arthroplasty is at least partly due to stress shielding produced by overly stiff metal implants. The ultimate success of this endeavor will depend on whether "stiffness matching" actually provides a significant benefit and whether serviceable composite implants can be produced at reasonable cost.

13.5.1.2 Hydroxyapatite

The mineral phase of bone—calcium hydroxyapatite (HAP)—has a complex hexagonal crystal structure made up of calcium, phosphorus, oxygen, and hydroxyl ions. It occurs as extremely fine crystals in bone and teeth and as much larger crystals of inorganic origin in nature. There is fairly convincing evidence that synthetic HAP, when implanted in a favorable (i.e., osteogenic) environment, can serve as a substrate for new bone formation and that significant bonding of bone to this substrate can occur. This circumstance, therefore, opens up the possibility of direct bonding of bone to load-bearing implants. HAP is not only brittle but is a relatively weak ceramic, especially after prolonged exposure to water, to which it is not totally immune. For this reason, little consideration has been given to using it in bulk as a load-bearing implant. The application of HAP coatings to tough metal substrates has received extensive development effort and even some commercial exposure, however. The success of these attempts depends on the manufacturer's ability to produce ceramic-metal bonding that is strong enough and durable enough for orthopaedic purposes. Prototype implants with HAP coatings have, so far, failed to achieve clinical acceptance.

13.5.2 Metals

As discussed in section 13.4.3, metals are generally strong, ductile, and chemically reactive. Most are far stronger than any polymer, and their ductility means that unanticipated catastrophic failure is a much rarer occurrence for metals than for ceramics. In fact, this combination of strength and ductility has made metal the material of choice for complex-loading (tensile) applications since the Bronze Age. As with most things in life, this very fortunate circumstance comes at a price, and the price in this case is that metals, because of their chemical reactivity, must always be protected from attack by the environment, particularly aqueous environments like that encountered in vivo. Fortunately, many metals, including all those used for orthopaedic implants, develop a natural protection against such attack. This is called passivation and is discussed in depth in chapter 15.

13.5.2.1 Crystal Structure

In Sections 13.4.1 to 13.4.3 we pointed out that the atoms of most solids tend to maximize the number of bonds with nearest neighbors and to minimize their energies by adopting arrangements that represent a high density of packing. Such dense packing is favored by the formation of crystals in which the atoms are arranged in orderly patterns that repeat in three dimensions. This is, in fact, the definition of a crystal. These structures can be represented by a small collection of spheres (in three-dimensional models) or circles (in two-dimensional drawings) called *unit cells* (figure 13.3). Unit cells possess all the geometric properties (i.e., symmetries) of the actual crystal and show the relationship of each atom to its neighbors. In fact, a model of a crystal could be generated by stacking up unit cells. Some 85% of all elemental metals crystallize in one of three densely packed structures: face-centered cubic (FCC; figure 13.3.a), hexagonal close-packed (HCP; figure 13.3b),

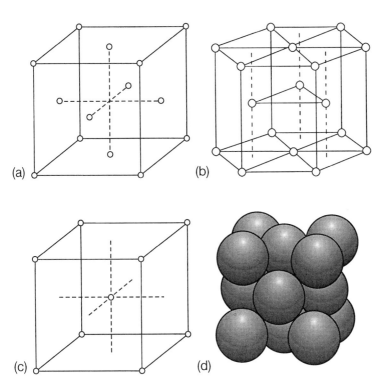

Figure 13.3. *(a)* Exploded view of face-centered cubic (FCC) unit cell. Although not obvious, an assembly of several of these unit cells will reveal the fact that each atom is surrounded by 12 nearest (contacting) neighbors. *(b)* Exploded view of hexagonal close-packed (HCP) unit cell. Each atom in this structure has 12 nearest neighbors. *(c)* Exploded view of body-centered cubic (BCC) unit cell. Each atom has eight nearest neighbors. *(d)* Unexploded view of an FCC unit cell showing the atoms in contact with their nearest neighbors.

and body-centered cubic (BCC; figure 13.3c). In both the FCC and HCP structures, each atom is in contact with 12 nearest neighbors, which is the densest packing possible with spheres of uniform size. When actual balls are packed in this configuration, they will occupy 74% of the volume available. In the BCC structure, each atom is in contact with only eight nearest neighbors. Surprisingly, this arrangement gives a packing density of 68%, which is only slightly less than that of the FCC and HCP structures. Note that the depiction of these crystal structures (figure 13.3) shows the atoms as small circles connected by lines. This exploded view makes it easier to visualize the whole structure in three dimensions. Keep in mind, however, that, in actual crystals, the atoms touch their nearest neighbors, as shown in figure 13.3.d.

13.5.2.2 Microstructure

When a molten metal is cooled to its solidification temperature, microscopic crystallites (i.e., crystal nuclei) form and then grow by the addition of more atoms from the melt. This growth continues until the crystals impinge on each other, and all the liquid has been consumed. At this point, the solid consists of many small, tightly packed crystals or grains separated by grain boundaries. The only thing that changes in crossing a grain boundary is the orientation of the crystals (figure 13.4).

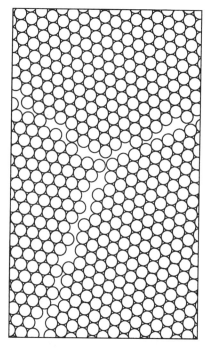

Figure 13.4. Two-dimensional model of three grain boundaries showing the change in orientation of the close-packed direction that occurs at each boundary. Notice also that about a one-atom diameter is required to reestablish order once the boundary has been crossed.

The grain boundaries themselves are regions of crystal imperfection and high energy and are only one or two atoms thick. This imperfection notwithstanding, the bonding across grain boundaries is very strong, and metals do not fail at grain boundaries except at high temperatures or in certain corrosive environments.

Solidification generally involves the formation of millions of nuclei per cubic centimeter of molten metal, so the grains in polycrystalline solids are typically 1–100 μm in diameter. For this reason, a microscope must be used to resolve the grain structure of metals. Because metals are opaque to visible light, a special reflecting or metallurgical microscope must be used (figure 13.5a). In this instrument, light is first reflected from the surface of the half-silvered prism, through the objective lens, and onto the polished surface of the metal. It is then reflected into the microscope through the prism and into the ocular lens. If the surface of the specimen is merely polished, it acts like a mirror, and the microscope image consists of nothing more than a bright spot. To observe the actual microstructure of the specimen, one must expose the polished surface to a mildly corrosive medium, often a dilute acid, called an *etch*. A properly chosen etch will attack the grain boundaries preferentially because they are regions of high energy and are, therefore, more reactive than the rest of the grain. The groove formed at the grain boundary scatters the incident light (figure 13.5b), and the result is that the grain boundary appears as a dark line in the microscope image. Figure 13.6 is a photomicrograph of the grain structure of a stainless steel sample. The microstructure of metals plays an important role in determining strength and corrosion resistance.

13.5.2.3 Alloys

Although all metals can be produced as pure elements, most structural applications use mixtures of two or more elements because they are generally much stronger than pure elements. These mixtures—called alloys—are usually created by adding the desired elements to the host metal in the molten state; that is, liquid metal solutions are formed in which the host (principal constituent) is the solvent, and the additions are the solutes. Upon cooling and solidification, crystallites of the solvent form and grow, with the solute atoms usually substituting randomly for some of the solvent atoms in the lattice sites of the solvent crystal. For example, the stainless steels used for orthopaedic implants (austenitic stainless steels) are alloys of iron, chromium, and nickel, in

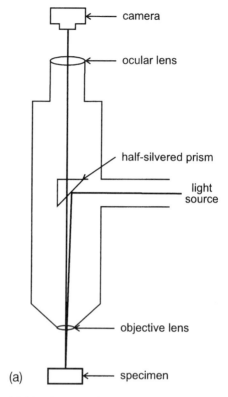

Figure 13.5. *(a)* Metallurgical (reflecting) microscope showing how the light beam enters the device, is reflected downward by the half-silvered prism, goes through the objective lens, and is reflected off the polished surface of the metallic specimen. It then passes upward through the objective lens again, through the prism, and through the ocular lens. When focused, a magnified image of the surface is projected onto the film of the camera. *(b)* Cross-sectional view of a metallographic specimen showing grooving at the grain boundary caused by etching. Light hitting the sides of the groove is scattered, causing the boundary to appear dark in the microscope image.

which the chromium and nickel atoms substitute for iron in the face-centered cubic lattice of the iron (figure 13.7). Note that all three of these alloying constituents are metals, and their atoms are very nearly the same size. In fact, the nickel and chromium atomic radii differ by only $\frac{1}{4}$ of 1%, and the iron radius is larger by only 1.2%. Thus, these

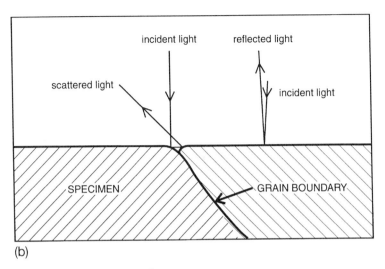

(b)

Figure 13.5. (continued)

Figure 13.6. Microstructure of wrought and annealed 316L stainless steel, showing grain boundaries and inclusions. The grains are approximately equiaxed (that is, have the same diameter in all directions), and the average grain diameter is approximately 140 μm. Magnification 100×. (Photomicrograph courtesy of Howmedica Inc., Rutherford, N.J.)

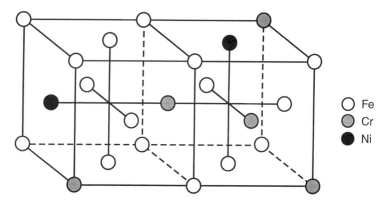

Figure 13.7. Crystal structure of implant-grade stainless steel showing chromium (Cr) and nickel (Ni) atoms substituted for iron (Fe) atoms on the FCC lattice.

elements enjoy wide ranges of solubility in each other. At the other extreme are the nonmetallic elements, principally oxygen, nitrogen, hydrogen, and carbon, whose atoms are small enough to fit into the open spaces, or interstices, of the metallic crystal lattices (figure 13.8). These are called interstitial alloying elements, and they are of great importance in many alloy systems, including all those used in orthopaedic implants.

In general, more solute can be dissolved in the solvent in the liquid phase than in the solid solution. If too much solute is added to the molten solution, two types of crystallites will form during solidification: one that is rich in the solvent and has the solvent-crystal structure and one that is rich in solute and has a different crystal structure. When solidification is complete, the resulting solid is a two-phase alloy consisting of a mixture of the two types of grains. Those with the solvent-crystal structure are usually identified as the α phase, and those with the different structure are labeled with a later letter in the Greek alphabet (e.g., β, γ, etc.). Both the titanium- and cobalt-based alloys used for orthopaedic implants are two-phase alloys (see chapter 14).

13.5.2.4 Strengthening of Alloys

Large single crystals of very pure elements are extremely weak. In laboratory testing they have been shown to have yield strengths as low as

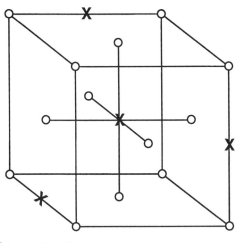

X interstitial site

Figure 13.8. FCC crystal structure showing the locations of some interstitial sites.

0.1–1.0 MPa, compared to 200–1,500 MPa for commercial orthopaedic alloys. A variety of mechanisms for strengthening metals are available to metallurgical engineers. Three of these are discussed here.

ALLOYING. When atoms of an alloying element are added to the crystal lattice of a solvent metal, the fit is never perfect; the solute atom is either a little too large or a little too small for the lattice site it must occupy. This size difference produces local strain (dilation or contraction) in the lattice. The greater the size difference, the greater the strain. This local strain in turn interferes with the local rearrangement of atoms necessary for plastic deformation; thus the metal's resistance to plastic deformation (i.e., its yield strength) increases as the amount of solute increases and as the atomic size difference increases. Although this happens with all alloy additions, it is particularly pronounced where interstitial additions are involved. In fact, the atoms of the interstitial elements (O, N, C, and H) are considerably larger than the interstitial sites can accommodate, causing large local strains to be produced when these elements are present. As an example, the yield strength of nominally pure titanium doubles if the oxygen content increases from

0.1 weight percent to 0.5 weight percent. Carbon is responsible for similar strengthening in steels (i.e., alloys of iron and carbon).

WORK HARDENING.   If a metal specimen is plastically deformed in a tensile test but unloaded before it breaks, it will exhibit an elevated yield strength upon reloading. This strengthening or work hardening is a result of permanent local strains that build up in the grains during plastic deformation. In commercial practice, metal parts are often exposed to forging (hammering or pressing) or rolling. When done at room temperature, this practice is called cold working, and it can easily elevate the strength of a metal by a factor of two or more. Such cold work reduces the ductility, however, and the forging process must be stopped at some point, or the part will fail by brittle fracture. If the cold-worked part is heated to a high enough temperature, all the effects of cold working can be completely reversed, and the material returns to its original soft, ductile condition. This heating process is called annealing. Parts are often formed by alternate cold forging (or rolling) and annealing. In this way, a cast block (ingot) a meter in diameter can be reduced to sheet or wire only a few tenths of a millimeter thick. It is also possible to conduct the forging or rolling operation at or near the annealing temperature so that the plastic deformation and annealing processes occur simultaneously. Naturally, this is called hot working. By controlling the amount of residual cold work in the finished piece, a wide range of strengths and ductilities can be achieved for an alloy of a given composition. This is the reason that tables of properties often show a range of strengths for a given metal alloy.

GRAIN SIZE.   Each grain in a metal sample is a small crystal that must undergo deformation commensurate with the overall deformation of the part as a whole. When one grain deforms, all the adjacent grains must deform in just the right way so that openings (i.e., voids) do not form at the boundaries between them. This cooperative deformation requires a higher applied stress than would comparable amounts of deformation in a large, single crystal. The result is that the existence of grain boundaries in a polycrystal is itself a potent strengthening agent, and the smaller the grain size, the greater the strengthening effect. The processes of hot working or cold working followed by annealing can actually reduce the grain size from that occurring in the original cast ingot. In fact, grain refinement is one of the main reasons thermomechanical processing is performed. This grain-size effect is further enhanced in two-phase alloys if the grains of the secondary phase are much harder than those of the primary phase. Manufacturers take advantage of all these mechanisms when producing metal alloys for orthopaedic implants.

13.5.3 Polymers

The third class of material used for structural applications is polymers. Discussion of the structure-property relationship in polymers usually begins with the polymer molecule. Note that the concept of a molecule was not involved when analyzing the structure of the other classes of solid materials. For instance, in crystalline sodium chloride, there are no identifiable Na-Cl pairs. In fact, earlier we emphasized the fact that each ion is associated equally with six nearest neighbors. One might even argue that the whole sodium chloride crystal constitutes one molecule in the solid state. The same sort of picture emerges for crystalline solids with covalent bonding. For example, silicon carbide is a very strong solid with covalent Si-C bonds and the diamond crystal structure. Going even further, the concept of a molecule must be abandoned entirely when one looks at metal crystals.

In considering the internal structure of organic polymers, however, it is useful to return to the molecular concept. In these materials, two of the covalent bonds are required to join the carbon atoms to form the polymer chain. If the two remaining bond sites are occupied by monovalent species such as hydrogen or chlorine, the chain can have no side branches or cross-links. In this case, the chain is linear and constitutes a true molecule with a measurable molecular weight. The bonding between chains, however, is weak, and the resulting solid is soft. It can be melted and resolidified at a relatively low temperature, and the individual molecules can be dispersed in solution by suitable solvents. The mechanical properties of these polymers depend on the length of the molecules, their degree of entanglement or organization, the size and nature of side groups, and the stiffness of the chain. In some linear polymers like polyethylene, the chains can be folded back upon themselves in orderly three-dimensional arrangements that constitute regions of true crystallinity in a matrix of randomly entangled (amorphous) material. In other linear polymers such as the polymethylmethacrylate (PMMA) used in bone cement, the structure is completely amorphous.

If some of the carbon atoms in the principal chain are covalently bonded to polyvalent side groups, particularly other carbon atoms, the polymer chains will start to exhibit branching or cross-linking. As these structural features increase, the strength and thermal stability of the polymer increase, but again the concept of molecularity becomes blurred. Obviously, manipulation of these many structural variables can give rise to polymers with a wide variety of properties. The interplay of these structure-property relationships is discussed in some detail in chapter 16.

Q13: Clinical Question (Summary)

Dr. Curmudgeon dropped a slippery ceramic femoral head onto the operating-room floor, where it shattered. Was the ceramic head defective? If not, could something so brittle be expected to function as a hip replacement?

A13: Clinical Answer

Ceramic is a very brittle material, but it is also very strong. As discussed in Section 13.5.1, it is very likely that an unusually large defect was present in the ball that Dr. Curmudgeon dropped. The stresses developed on striking the floor were great enough to trigger catastrophic growth of this crack. It would be impossible to know this for sure without examination of the fracture surfaces, but it is possible that Dr. Curmudgeon inadvertently did the patient a favor!

Additional Reading

Bhambri S, Gilbertson L: Zirconia Femoral Heads. Technical Monograph 97–2100–18. Zimmer, Warsaw, Ind., 1996.

Cooke FW: Ceramics in orthopaedic surgery. *Clin Orthop Rel Res* 276:135, 1992.

Dumbleton JHH, Black J: *An Introduction to Orthopaedic Materials.* Charles C Thomas, Springfield, Ill., 1975.

Fuller RA, Rosen JJ: Materials for medicine. *Sci Am* 255(4): 118, 1986.

Hydroxyapatite: Key Facts and Issues. Technical Monograph 6090–0-001–1. Howmedica, Rutherford, N.J., 1994.

Liedl GL: The science of materials. *Sci Am* 255(4): 127, 1986.

Park JB: *Biomaterials Science and Engineering.* Plenum Press, New York, 1984.

Pauling L: *The Nature of the Chemical Bond and the Structure of Molecules and Crystals.* Cornell Univ. Press, Ithaca, N. Y., 1960.

Ratner BD, Hoffman AS, Schoen, FJ, Lemons JE: *Biomaterials Science.* Academic Press, New York, 1996.

von Recum AF, Ed.: *Handbook of Biomaterials Evaluation.* Macmillan, New York, 1986.

14

Orthopaedic Alloys

CLINICAL SCENARIO: WHICH IS BETTER — TITANIUM OR COBALT CHROME?

At the time that Charley Davidson had his fractured tibia treated, it was customary to treat such fractures with an intramedullary rod if the soft tissue wound was not too severe. Tibial rods were customarily made of cobalt-chrome alloy and were quite serviceable, but recently a trend to making such rods out of titanium had developed. Metal is metal, is it not, and why would one type be any better or worse than another?

In chapter 13 we saw that metals are the preferred materials for implant devices subjected to high in vivo stresses because they combine good strength with resistance to brittle fracture. We also learned that alloys are used for these applications rather than pure metals because alloys can be prepared with much higher strengths. In chapter 15 we see how considerations of corrosion resistance have influenced the selection of particular alloys for implant applications. In this chapter we examine the composition, structure, and mechanical properties of the alloys used for orthopaedic implants. In pursuing this objective, we remind the reader that the strength of a given alloy does not depend on its composition alone but is also a function of its fabrication history and microstructure.

■ 14.1 STAINLESS STEELS

The term *steel* refers to a vast family of alloys based on iron and carbon. By adjusting the carbon content and the thermomechanical processing of these alloys, we can produce an extremely wide variety of mechanical properties. If chromium is added as an alloying element in amounts greater than 12%, the usual atmospheric corrosion (i.e., rusting), typical of iron alloys, is suppressed. These alloys are called stainless steels, and even this subset includes a number of specific alloy compositions. The alloy used for virtually all surgical implants carries the alphanumeric designation 316L, which indicates that nickel and molybdenum have been added as well as chromium. The L indicates that the carbon content is held at a low level—below 0.03% by weight (w/o) for improved corrosion resistance. A list of all the major and minor alloying additions specified* for 316L stainless steel is presented in table 14.1. The molybdenum and nickel are added for the specific purpose of increasing the corrosion resistance of the alloy against chloride-containing solutions such as the physiological environment. (These corrosion considerations are discussed in more detail in chapter 15.)

The equilibrium crystal structure of most iron alloys at room temperature is body-centered cubic (BCC), called ferrite, whereas the face-centered cubic (FCC) structure called austenite exists at elevated temperatures. The addition of nickel in amounts above 8 w/o not only enhances the corrosion resistance of 316L stainless steel but stabilizes the FCC structure at room temperature. For this reason, 316L stainless steel is said to be an austenitic stainless steel. Because plastic deformation is easier in the FCC than in the BCC structure, 316L stainless steel is relatively weak and ductile for a steel. This tendency is reinforced by holding the carbon content below 0.03 w/o. At higher levels, carbon would be a potent strengthening agent. No precipitates or second phases are formed during the processing of 316L stainless steel, so the microstructure is that of a simple, single-phase alloy (figure 13.6). An effort is made to ensure that the grains are as uniform in size as possible and that the average grain diameter is less than about 100 μm. This provides for some strengthening of the alloy by virtue of the small grain-size effect. In addition, great care is taken to minimize the pres-

---

*The composition microstructure, properties, evaluation, and testing of commercial devices and materials are established in series of detailed specifications developed and voluntarily adhered to by manufacturers. The process of establishing these specifications is administered by the American Society for Testing and Materials (ASTM), W. Conshohocken, Pennsylvania. The ASTM Committee F4 is responsible for Specification of Medical and Surgical Materials and Devices. Similar international standards are established by the International Standards Organization (ISO).

Table 14.1 Chemical composition of 316L stainless steel[a]

Element	Composition (%)
Carbon	0.03 max
Chromium	17–19
Nickel	13–15
Molybdenum	2–3
Iron	Balance

[a]From ASTM specification F138–92

ence of ceramic inclusions, such as oxide, sulfide, and silicate particles that may be entrapped in the metal during melting and pouring. Such inclusions act as local stress raisers that reduce both strength and ductility.

Because of the low carbon content and simple microstructure annealed, 316L stainless steel has the lowest yield strength and greatest ductility of the three standard orthopaedic-implant alloys. In order to increase its strength, 316L stainless steel is often used in the partially cold-worked condition. The mechanical properties of this and other alloys are presented in table 14.2. The properties of compact bone and bone cement are also included for comparison. The alloy strength values given in this table are the minimum values required by the relevant specifications. The actual strength values for real samples of these alloys are usually greater by 30% or more.

■ **14.2 COBALT-BASED ALLOYS**

In the 1930s cobalt-based alloys were pressed into service as orthopaedic-implant materials because they were more corrosion resistant than the stainless steels available at the time. At temperatures above 420°C, pure cobalt assumes the FCC crystal structure, which is designated as the alpha form. Below this temperature, cobalt transforms slowly to the hexagonal close-packed (HCP), or beta, form; however,

Table 14.2 Minimum mechanical properties of implant alloys, compact bone, and bone cement

Material	Condition	Modulus (GPa)	Yield strength (MPa)	Ultimate tensile strength (MPa)	Elongation (%)	ASTM Spec.
316L	Annealed	190	170	480	40	F138
316L	Cold worked	190	310–690	655–860	28–12	F138
Co-Cr-Mo	Cast	210	450	655	8	F75
Co-Cr-Mo	Forged and annealed	210	827	1172	12	F799
Co-Cr-W-Ni	Forged and annealed	210	379	896	30–45	F90
Ti 6Al/4V	Forged and annealed	113	795–827	860–900	10	F136
Bone	Compact	12–24[a]	–	50–160[a]	0	–
Bone cement	PMMA	2.2	–	30–45[b]	0	F451

[a]Depends strongly on direction of testing

[b]Experimental results, strength values are not included in the ASTM specification

in the highly alloyed materials used in implants, the transformation is so sluggish that the alpha form persists at room temperature.

14.2.1 Cast Alloys

Typically the cobalt-based implant alloys contain 20%–30% chromium, which is the primary reason for their excellent corrosion resistance. In the original implants of the 1930s, the alloy was processed directly into components by casting the molten metal into ceramic molds. Upon removal from the mold, the components required only surface finishing and polishing to produce a final product. This method of fabrication was economical, but the grain size produced was very large due to the slow cooling in the mold. In addition, a very high carbon content was required for increased strength. Upon cooling to room temperature, much of the carbon precipitated as carbides of chromium, cobalt, and molybdenum. The combination of large, as cast, alpha grains and large second-phase precipitates impaired both the strength and the corrosion resistance of these components. The composition of the casting alloy (ASTM F75) is given in table 14.3, and a typical, as cast microstructure is shown in figure 14.1.

14.2.2 Wrought Alloys

As the use of cast implants increased and long-term clinical experience accumulated, especially with heavily loaded prostheses, fatigue

Table 14.3 Composition of cobalt-based implant alloys

| | Type (ASTM Spec) | | | |
Component	F75 (Cast)	F799 (Wrought)	F90 (Wrought)	F562 (MP35N)
Carbon	0.35% max.	0.35% max.	0.15% max.	0.025% max.
Chromium	30%	30%	20%	20%
Molybdenum	6%	6%	0%	10%
Nickel	1%	1%	10%	35%
Tungsten	—	—	15%	—
Cobalt	Balance	Balance	Balance	Balance

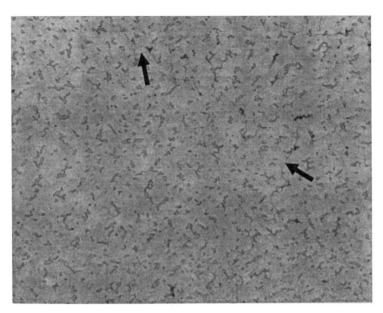

Figure 14.1. Microstructure of cast cobalt-chromium-molybdenum (Co-Cr-Mo) alloy (F75) showing very large alpha grains (only parts of several grains are included) with large carbide particles throughout grains and at grain boundaries. Arrows indicate grain boundaries. Magnification 100×. (Photomicrograph courtesy of Howmedica Inc., Rutherford, N.J.)

failures became a matter of concern. In response to this challenge, manufacturers began to produce implants from wrought material. Instead of casting the alloy directly in the final component shape, large blocks, or ingots, were cast. These were subjected to forging (plastic deformation) and heating steps that resulted in bar stock with a much finer grain size and a fine dispersion of second-phase particles. These well-dispersed, fine particles are very hard and contribute substantially to the strength of this alloy. Figure 14.2 shows a typical microstructure of this alloy, and table 14.2 shows that the yield and ultimate tensile strengths have nearly doubled as compared to the cast alloy. This remarkable achievement can be better appreciated by referring to figure 14.3, which is a graphical presentation of the strength data. In addition to the gain in strength, the ductility, corrosion resistance, and fatigue resistance were all improved. On the other hand, the

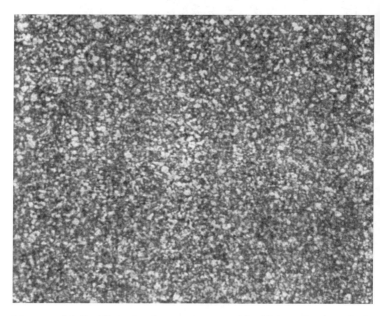

Figure 14.2. Microstructure of wrought high-carbon cobalt-chromium-molybdenum (Co-Cr-Mo) alloy (F799) showing fine dispersion of carbides in small-grained α matrix. Magnification 200×. (Photomicrograph courtesy of Howmedica Inc., Rutherford, N.J.)

production of bar stock meant that components had to be fabricated entirely by difficult and expensive machining processes. The wrought alloy has the same chemical composition as the cast material, but a separate ASTM specification, F799, has been developed to cover the improved mechanical properties available.

A slightly different wrought cobalt alloy, F90, is also used for orthopaedic implants. This alloy has 10 w/o nickel and 15 w/o tungsten, but only 20 w/o chromium and 0.15 w/o carbon (table 14.3). These composition changes result in a microstructure of alpha grains with virtually no second-phase (carbide) precipitates. In the annealed condition, the absence of a fine carbide dispersion causes this alloy to have strength values even lower than the F75 cast alloy but with much higher ductility. Cold working, however, can increase the strength of this alloy to levels that exceed those of the F799 wrought alloy (see fig-

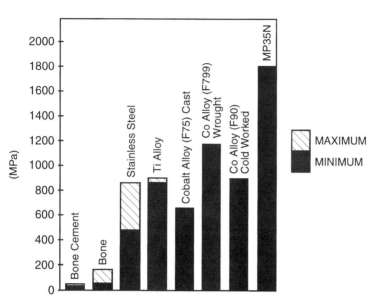

Figure 14.3. Ultimate tensile strength of selected materials and orthopaedic-implant alloys.

ure 14.3). It is more difficult and expensive to realize these advantages as compared to the fabrication of the F799 alloy, however.

Both the wrought alloys just described have cobalt contents greater than 50 w/o. An even more heavily alloyed material, called MP 35N, is also available. This alloy contains 20 w/o chromium, 35 w/o nickel, 10 w/o molybdenum, and only 35 w/o cobalt (table 14.3). After appropriate thermomechanical processing, this alloy has a multiphase microstructure—that is, both alpha (FCC) and beta (HCP) grains are present. The beta grains are very finely dispersed, and this alloy can achieve a tensile strength of 1,800 MPa in the cold-worked and heat-treated condition (figure 14.3).

14.2.3 Powder-Metal Alloys

Cobalt alloys with a fine grain size can be produced by a powder metallurgy technique that offers an alternative to the thermomechanical processing of large ingots. Alloy particles—powders—are produced by spraying, or atomizing, molten metal into a large chamber filled with a cold, low-pressure gas like argon. The tiny droplets that are formed cool and solidify as they fall to the bottom of the chamber. The particles are then separated according to size by sieving, and the finer particles are pressed in a closed die. The pressing is typically conducted at 1,100°C and 100 MPa of pressure for 1 hour. Because the pressurization is uniform over the surface of the part, this process is called hot isostatic pressing or HIP-ing. The final product of HIP-ing is fully dense with no porosity and is very close to the desired component shape, so only light finish machining is required. HIP-ed alloys can have a grain size smaller than 10 μm with very fine carbide particles, giving these materials exceptionally good mechanical properties.

An ingenious variation on these powder metallurgy alloys was developed in the late 1980s.* Small amounts of strong oxide formers—aluminum and lanthanum—were added to the conventional cobalt-chromium-molybdenum (Co-Cr-Mo) casting alloy (F75) just prior to atomization. The resulting powders contained an extremely fine dispersion of insoluble aluminum and lanthanum oxide particles. After HIP-ing, these oxide particles stabilize the grain size at less than 20 μm. The process for producing this material is called gas atomized-dispersion strengthening, or GADS. This material was developed primarily for use in porous-coated prostheses. The process of applying porous coatings tends to degrade the fatigue resistance of the substrate metal, but, as we shall see in the last section of this chapter, the fine oxide dispersion in the GADS alloys offsets this effect to a substantial degree.

■ 14.3 TITANIUM ALLOYS

Titanium alloys first became available for service as surgical implant materials in the mid1960s, much later than the stainless steels and cobalt alloys. The initial reason for their consideration was their exceptional corrosion resistance, including resistance to chloride-containing solutions, and the absence of cobalt, chromium, and nickel from their composition. This latter consideration arises from the persistent suspicion that one or more of the components of the older alloys may be re-

---

*Howmedica Inc., Rutherford, New Jersey

sponsible for an allergic reaction similar to metal sensitivity in some patients. Titanium alloys remain the materials of choice for patients with a history of severe metal sensitivity. At a somewhat later date, an additional potential advantage for titanium alloys was recognized. The stiffness, or elastic modulus, of titanium and its alloys is only about half that of the other implant alloys (figure 14.4). This means that bone atrophy due to stress shielding of the proximal femur should be lessened if a titanium-alloy prosthesis is used rather than one made of stainless steel or a cobalt alloy. The complicating and probably overriding effect of wear-particle-induced osteolysis in total hip arthroplasty has obscured the potential benefit of lower stiffness implants, however, and so far it has not been possible to demonstrate that a reduced modulus really offers a clear-cut clinical advantage. This uncertainty not withstanding, titanium alloys have achieved wide acceptance as implant materials in orthopaedics because of their exceptional corrosion resistance and superior biocompatibility.

Modulus of Elasticity of Selected Materials

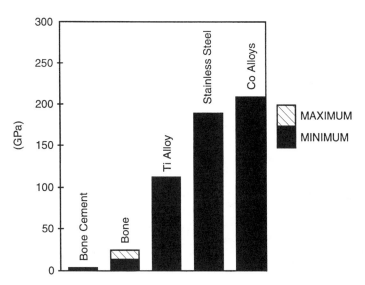

Figure 14.4. Modulus of elasticity of selected materials and orthopaedic implant alloys.

14.3.1 Structure of Titanium Alloys

As we saw with iron and cobalt, titanium exhibits two crystal structures: a BCC form called *beta* above 882°C and an HCP form called *alpha* from 882°C down to room temperature. The alloy most commonly used for implants contains 6% aluminum and 4% vanadium and is generally designated as Ti 6Al/4V. The aluminum tends to stabilize the alpha form, and the vanadium stabilizes the beta form. This composition was chosen specifically so that the competition between these effects would provide the possibility for these two phases to exist simultaneously at room temperature. The actual structure that is produced depends primarily on the temperatures at which the forging and annealing treatments are conducted. For the most part, air cooling of small parts like prosthesis components leads to a mixture of fine alpha and beta grains (figure 14.5) that provides tensile and fatigue properties comparable to those of the cobalt alloys (table 14.2 and figure 14.3).

An important concern in processing titanium and its alloys is the embrittling effect of unintentional additions of small interstitial atoms

Figure 14.5. Microstructure of titanium 6%Al-4%V alloy showing equiaxed alpha grains and a fine dispersion of beta grains.

(i.e., oxygen, nitrogen, hydrogen, and carbon). Oxygen and nitrogen, in particular, are absorbed from the air whenever titanium or its alloys are raised to elevated temperatures, so all high-temperature processing must be conducted in a vacuum or under a protective atmosphere of argon. The specification for the composition of implant-grade Ti 6Al/4V (ASTM F136; table 14.4) requires that the total interstitial content be less than 0.27%. This is designated as the extra low interstitial or ELI grade. Even with this low interstitial content, the ductility of this alloy in terms of elongation is only 10%.

By the end of the 1980s, titanium alloys with all beta structures were developed specifically for orthopaedic implant applications. They contain zirconium and large amounts of BCC elements (i.e., beta stabilizers), including niobium, molybdenum, and iron. These alloys are reported to be superior to Ti 6Al/4V in strength, ductility, toughness, and biocompatibility and to have greater resistance to wear and fatigue. They also have elastic moduli that are even lower than that of the Ti 6Al/4V alloy. It will be interesting to follow the clinical performance of these alloys if their use becomes more widespread over the next several years.

■ 14.4 WEAR OF IMPLANT ALLOYS

At one time or another, all three of the standard orthopaedic implant alloys have been used as articulating components in total-joint-replace-

Table 14.4 Composition of titanium alloys

Component	6Al/4V (ASTM, F136)
Interstitials	0.27% max.
Aluminum	5.5–6.5%
Vanadium	3.5–4.5%
Molybdenum	–
Zirconium	–
Iron	0.25% max.
Titanium	balance

ment systems. The rubbing action involved in this type of service gradually removes material from the surface of the component by a variety of mechanical processes known collectively as wear. At the present time, the majority of the wear debris released in total-joint systems comes from the polyethylene component, which is much softer than the metal counter face and wears at a much higher rate. Nonetheless, significant quantities of particles are also released from the metal side, particularly when the Ti 6Al/4V alloy is used. In fact, titanium-alloy particles are released in such abundance that the periarticular tissues can become extensively blackened. Note that all finely divided metal powders are black, whereas polyethylene particles imbedded in tissue are undetectable with the naked eye. Although it can be disconcerting to see titanium-blackened tissue at revision surgery, there is no clear evidence that these particles add appreciably to the problem of wear particle induced osteolysis, which is associated primarily with polyethylene wear debris. Metal wear debris will become a much greater concern in the future, however, if the renewed interest in metal-on-metal prostheses should lead to a resurgence in their clinical use. Laboratory studies in vitro indicate that the beta titanium alloys may be significantly more wear resistant than the alpha plus beta alloys. Nevertheless, their use in metal-on-metal articulations is contraindicated.

■ 14.5 FATIGUE OF IMPLANT ALLOYS

The advent of porous-coated prostheses, especially porous-coated femoral components for total hip replacement systems, has given rise to renewed concern about the fatigue resistance of implant alloys. The application of porous coatings to alloy substrates introduces two factors that increase fatigue susceptibility. The first is the creation of sharp notches where the beads or wires of the coating are fused to the substrate surface. These notches act as stress raisers that lower the apparent fatigue strength of the component. In response to this threat, some manufacturers have excluded the porous coatings from the surfaces that experience the greatest tensile stresses (i.e., the proximal lateral surface of femoral components). The second problem is that the porous coatings must be fused to the implant surface by prolonged exposure to elevated temperatures. This treatment, called sintering, causes the beads or wires to fuse firmly to the implant, but it also leads to large grains in both the cobalt-based alloys and the Ti 6Al/4V alloy. These large grains then serve to further reduce fatigue resistance. The GADS cobalt alloy with its oxide-particle-stabilized microstructures was specifically developed to counter this problem. It has also been shown that the beta titanium alloys have greater resistance to notch fatigue than the conventional alpha plus beta alloys.

Q14: CLINICAL QUESTION (SUMMARY)

At the time of Mr. Davidson's accident, tibial rods were customarily made of cobalt-chromium (Co-Cr) alloy, but recently there had been a trend toward making such rods out of titanium. Metal is metal, is it not, and why would one type be any better or worse than another?

A14: CLINICAL ANSWER

At this point, it should be clear that stainless steel is used primarily where its great ductility is of clinical value, but the cobalt- and titanium-based alloys are preferred for prostheses and other applications where high strength and long-term corrosion resistance are at a premium. The advantages of cobalt alloys are their high strength and fatigue resistance, especially when porous coatings are present; the advantages of the Ti 6Al/4V alloy are its exceptional corrosion resistance and biocompatibility. Recent improvements in both these alloy systems promise greatly improved performance in the not-too-distant future.

Additional Reading

Bardos DI: High strength Co-Cr-Mo alloy by hot isostatic pressing of powder. *Biomater Med Devices Artif Organs* 7(1):3, 1979.

Devine TM, Wulff, J: Cast vs. wrought Co-Cr surgical implant alloy. *J Biomed Mater Res* 9:151, 1975.

Implant Porous Coatings. Technical Monograph. Smith & Nephew Richards, Memphis, Tenn., 1995.

Laing PG, Galante JO, Lautenschlager E: Biomaterials: orthopaedic implants. In *Medical Devices.* CA Coceres, HT Yolken, RJ Jones, HR Piehler, Eds. ASTM STP 800, American Society for Testing and Materials, West Conshohocken, Pa., p. 74, 1983.

Levine DL: *The Effect of Material Stiffness on the Function of Cemented Tibial Trays: Ti-6Al-4V vs. Co-Cr Alloy*. Technical Monograph 97–2100–05. Zimmer, Inc., Warsaw, Ind., 1995.

Modular Femoral Head Taper Technology. Technical Monograph. Smith & Nephew Richards, Memphis, Tenn., 1995.

Pilliar RM: Modern metal processing for improved load-bearing surgical implants. *Biomaterials* 12:95, 1991.

Rostocker W, Chao EYS, Galante JO: Defects in failed stems of hip prostheses. *J Biomed Mater Res* 12:635, 1978.

Shetty R, Compton R, Kirkpatrick L, Kenyon R: *Properties of Porous Coatings Used in the Fabrication of Hip Prostheses.* Technical Monograph 97–2100–17. Zimmer, Inc., Warsaw, Ind., 1996.

TMSF: A Beta Titanium Alloy for Orthopaedic Implants. Technical Monograph 6260–5-002–0. Howmedica, Rutherford, N.J., 1996.

Yue S, Pilliar RM, Weatherly GC: The fatigue strength of porous-coated Ti6% AL-4%V implant alloys. *J Biomed Mater Res* 18:1043, 1984.

15

Corrosion in the Body

CLINICAL SCENARIO: USE OF A TITANIUM FEMORAL STEM WITH A COBALT-CHROMIUM HEAD

Continuing with the question concerning titanium, a further episode in the life of Dr. Curmudgeon bears repeating. Early in the development of total hip implants, the implants were available in just a few sizes and configurations, but as more and more different types of patients were operated on, more options were needed. Thus evolved the concept of modularity, which allowed different heads to be put together with different shaft configurations, neck lengths, and so on. Dr. Curmudgeon was not aware one day that, after he had placed a titanium shaft into the femoral canal, the scrub nurse had handed him a cobalt-chromium (Co-Cr) alloy femoral head of the appropriate size. Is the difference in the two metals likely to cause any problems, and, if so, what sort of problems should we expect?

In chapter 13 we discussed the fact that metals are the preferred materials for highly stressed orthopaedic implants because they combine good strength with the ability to plastically deform; in other words, metals and their alloys are tough. The free-electron model of metallic bonding provided an explanation of this unique combination of mechanical properties but also showed that metals are very chemically reactive compared to ceramics and polymers. Table 15.1 shows the heat that is released when some common metals react with oxygen to

Table 15.1   Heats of formation of selected metal oxides and CO_2

Metal	Compound	Heat of formation (kcal/mole)
Aluminum	Al_2O_3	−399.1
Chromium	Cr_2O_3	−269.7
Titanium	TiO_2	−218.0
Iron (3^+)	F_2O_3	−196.5
Magnesium	MgO	−143.8
Carbon (coal)	CO_2	−70 to −90
Zinc	ZnO	−83.2
Tin	SnO	−68.4
Iron (2^+)	FeO	−63.7
Nickel	NiO	−58.4
Cobalt	CoO	−57.2
Copper	CuO	−37.1
Silver	Ag_2O	−7.3
Gold	Au_2O_3	+19.3

form oxides. Those above carbon in the list are stable oxides indeed and, in fact, are always found in the combined state in nature. The heat of formation of the oxide is the energy that must be input in order to extract the elemental metal from its (oxide) ore. Thereafter, the metal is in a metastable condition just waiting for an opportunity to react with its environment and return to its lower-energy state. *When this return trip takes place slowly, near room temperature, and in the presence of an aqueous solution, it is called corrosion.* The purpose of this chapter is to explore the details of the corrosion process—how it occurs, how it is circumvented, and how it influences the use of metals in orthopaedics.

Before leaving Table 15.1, take a look at the elements at the bottom of the list. Note that these are a few metals (notably, silver, and gold) with relatively small (or even positive) heats of oxidation. These are called the noble metals because of their low reactivity; they can be found in nature (if one is lucky) in their elemental state. Dentists use these metals in small amounts in the body, but their high cost and relatively low strength make their use in orthopaedics impractical.

■ 15.1 ELECTROCHEMICAL CORROSION

Essentially all corrosion in the body is electrochemical in nature. If a metal rod or electrode is immersed in water, some of its atoms will go into solution as positive ions (i.e., cations), leaving behind some electrons so that the electrode becomes slightly negatively charged (figure 15.1):

$$M \rightarrow M^+ + e^-$$

As this process continues, the concentration of cations in solution increases, and the growing negative charge on the electrode begins to attract some of the cations back to the electrode:

$$M \leftarrow M^+ + e^-$$

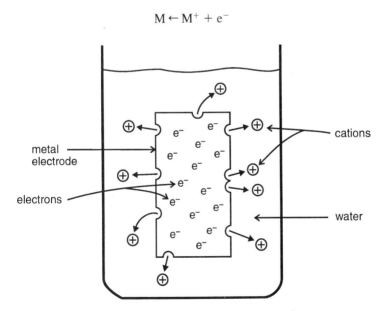

Figure 15.1. Metal electrode in water, showing dissolution of positive ions (cations) into solution and charging of the electrode due to retained electrons.

When the rate of the forward and reverse reactions becomes equal, that is, when dynamic equilibrium is established, the metal electrode will possess a certain charge. If the potential due to this charge is measured against some standard reference electrode, one will find that the potential difference is characteristic of the metal (figure 15.2). In general, the greater this potential for a given metal, the greater is its tendency to ionize and corrode. Table 15.2 is a list of these standard electrode potentials (SEP) for some metals of interest measured in a specific solution against a hydrogen standard electrode.

A comparison of table 15.2 with table 15.1 will show that the metals with the highest chemical reactivity tend to have the highest SEPs (e.g., Mg, Al, and Ti), and those with positive SEPs tend to be the least reactive. In general, the metals with the highest (most negative) SEP tend to be the most likely to corrode or to corrode the fastest in a given envi-

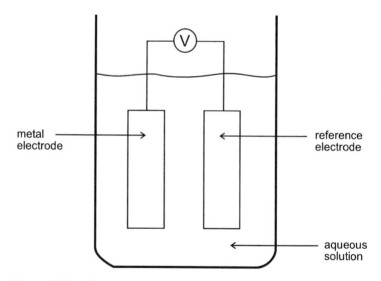

Figure 15.2. The use of a reference electrode to determine the relative potential of a metal immersed in an aqueous solution of its ions. If the metal electrode is in equilibrium with a one-molal solution of its own ions and if the reference electrode is a so-called hydrogen electrode in equilibrium with a one-molal solution of hydrogen ions, the resulting potential will be the Standard Electrode Potential (SEP) for that metal.

Table 15.2 Standard electrode potentials for some selected metals

	Metal	Ion	Electrode Potential (volts)
Anodic	Sodium	Na^{1+}	−2.71
	Magnesium	Mg^{2+}	−2.38
	Aluminum	Al^{3+}	−1.67
	Titanium	Ti^{2+}	−1.63
	Vanadium	V^{2+}	−1.20
	Zinc	Zn^{2+}	−0.76
	Chromium	Cr^{2+}	−0.56
	Iron	Fe^{2+}	−0.44
	Cobalt	Co^{2+}	−0.28
	Nickel	Ni^{2+}	−0.25
	Tin	Sn^{2+}	−0.14
	Hydrogen[a]	H^{1+}	0.00
	Copper	Cu^{2+}	+0.34
	Silver	Ag^{1+}	+0.80
	Platinum	Pt^{2+}	+1.20
Cathodic	Gold	Au^{1+}	+1.80

[a]Standard reference electrode

ronment. Note that the SEPs listed in table 15.2 were determined for pure elements under very carefully controlled conditions. Similar rankings have been developed for standard commercial alloys (including those of interest to orthopaedists) in a variety of solutions. These constitute galvanic series, and the one developed for seawater (Figure 15.3) is considered to be a reasonable approximation of the conditions encountered by implant alloys in the body. Notice that the galvanic potentials for a given alloy are shown with a range of values. This is because the composition, processing, and surface finish of commercial specimens can vary to some degree, and this effects their reactivity.

STANDARD ELECTRODE POTENTIAL (Volts)

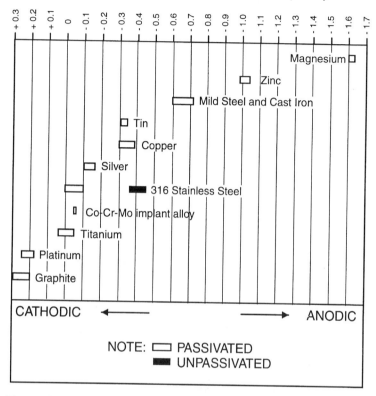

Figure 15.3. Galvanic series for selected metals and alloys in flowing (aerated) seawater. *Adapted from:* Laque FL: *Marine Corrosion: Causes and Prevention.* Wiley, New York, 1975, p. 179, figure 6–1.

■ 15.2 ELECTRODE REACTIONS

So far we have considered only circumstances where the corrosion process released ions that went into solution and remained there. This is not what usually happens in real life. Consider the situation of a zinc electrode in water. As the zinc ions go into solution, the hydrogen ions will be attracted to the electrode by the growing negative charge on it. (Remember there are 10^{-7} hydrogen ions present per mole of pure water; that is what pH 7 means.) Upon adsorption of a hydrogen ion on the surface, an electron is transferred to that ion, and the charge on the electrode is reduced while a neutral hydrogen atom is formed:

$$e^- + H^+ \rightarrow H$$

Eventually the hydrogen atoms combine to form hydrogen molecules that in turn coalesce to form hydrogen gas bubbles that rise to the surface of the cell and escape. Because this process tends to reduce the negative charge accumulating on the electrode, it keeps the corrosion of the zinc going. If the hydrogen ion concentration is increased, say by adding a little hydrochloric acid, the reaction accelerates because there are now plenty of H^+ ions available. Vigorous bubbling of the escaping hydrogen occurs. This same sort of reaction occurs for many metals (Fe, Al, Mg, etc.) in a variety of acids. In general, decreasing the pH of a solution will increase the rate of corrosion of metals. An important exception can occur in certain circumstances. If the neutral hydrogen atoms fail to combine into hydrogen molecules or if the hydrogen molecules fail to form bubbles that escape, the neutral species adsorbed on the surface can insulate the metal from the corrosive environment and actually slow down the corrosion process. This phenomenon is called polarization, and it can have a major influence on corrosion processes.

Let us next consider the corrosion of iron in a neutral (i.e., pH 7) solution saturated with oxygen, such as interstitial fluid or seawater. The following reaction occurs:

$$2Fe + 2H_2O + O_2 \rightarrow 2Fe^{2+} + 4(OH)^{1-} \rightarrow 2Fe\,(OH)_2$$

The final corrosion product—ferrous hydroxide ($Fe(OH)_2$)—is relatively insoluble in water and tends to precipitate out of solution as loose flakes. In addition, it reacts further with the oxygen in the water as follows:

$$2\,Fe\,(OH)_2 + H_2O + \tfrac{1}{2}O_2 \rightarrow 2\,Fe\,(OH)_3$$

The mixture of $Fe(OH)_2$ and $Fe(OH)_3$ is reddish brown in color, and you would immediately recognize it as rust. Note that the loose flakes do not adhere to the metal surface, and rusting usually proceeds unabated until the component fails due to reduced cross section or is completely consumed.

■ 15.3 DISSIMILAR METALS OR GALVANIC CORROSION

If specimens of two different metals are placed in contact with each other and are submerged in an aqueous solution, a corrosion couple or galvanic couple is created (figure 15.4). The more active metal will undergo corrosion, while a different chemical reaction will take place on the surface of the less active metal. *The corroding metal, the one releasing ions into solution and becoming negatively charged, is called the anode, and the other is the cathode.* The chemical reaction at the anode is the anodic reaction:

$$M \rightarrow e^- + M^+$$

The reaction at the cathode is, of course, the cathodic reaction.

A variety of cathodic reactions is possible depending mainly on the composition of the electrolyte. The anodic reaction is an oxidation reaction for the obvious reason that the generation of positive ions from the metal of the anode is a step toward returning that metal to its low-

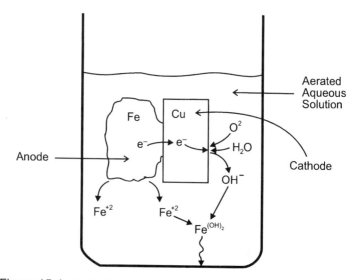

Figure 15.4. A dissimilar metal (galvanic) couple of iron and copper in an aerated water solution like seawater or interstitial fluid.

energy oxidized state. The reaction at the cathode is a reducing reaction. *A basic rule governing galvanic corrosion is that the rate of oxidation at the anode must equal the rate of reduction at the cathode.* In other words, the electrons released in the anodic reaction must all be consumed in the cathodic reaction if the reaction is to be ongoing.

Consider what happens if a zinc anode is coupled with a noble metal cathode like platinum. In this simple case the cathode reaction will be

$$e^- + H^+ \rightarrow H$$

because the noble metal itself is inert in this environment. This coupling will have the effect of greatly accelerating both reactions, however, because the large cathode area provides a great opportunity for hydrogen-ion neutralization. In addition, if platinum is used, it will catalyze the formation of hydrogen molecules.

Refer to the galvanic series in figure 15.3 to observe that there is about a 1.22-V difference between the zinc and the platinum, which is the driving force for the accelerated corrosion of the zinc. In general, whenever dissimilar metals are in contact in a saline solution, the more electronegative one will become the anode (will corrode), and the voltage difference is an indication of how fast the corrosion reaction will proceed.

Let us consider what happens when a more complex cathode reaction is involved. If an iron sample is coupled with a piece of copper, the iron will be the anode, and the potential difference will be about 0.18 V (figure 15.4). The iron will release iron ions into solution, but the copper will not; that is, the copper will be protected (figure 15.4). The cathodic reaction will be

$$O_2 + 2 H_2O + 4 e^- \rightarrow 4 (OH)^-$$

The cathodic reaction then involves the reduction of O_2 to OH^-, which supplies hydroxyl ions for the formation of ferrous and ferric hydroxide, as we saw earlier. To repeat, the copper provides a substrate for the cathode reaction but does not take part itself. Thus, the copper is protected from corrosion. This phenomenon is sometimes utilized in industrial situations such as the coupling of magnesium sacrificial anodes to steel oil well towers standing in seawater. Here the rapid corrosion of the magnesium protects the load-bearing structure, steel (iron), from attack. This technique has not found an application in surgical implants, however, probably due to the fact that ions of the anodic element would be released into the physiologic environment, which would be undesirable.

■ 15.4 PASSIVATION

We are now ready to reveal the secret of how some of the most reactive metals (i.e., metals with the highest standard electrode potentials and the highest heats of oxide formation, for example, titanium, aluminum, vanadium, and chromium) can be used in implant alloys with seeming immunity from corrosion. When these metals are placed in an oxidizing atmosphere, which may be just ambient air, they do in fact oxidize rapidly, but the oxide formed remains tenaciously bonded to the surface of the metal as a thin film. This film isolates the metal from the atmosphere, and the metal ions must migrate through the film by diffusion— a very slow process at room temperature—to gain access to the environment. As oxidation continues, the film gets thicker and thicker, and diffusion takes longer and longer until it comes to a complete halt as far as the loss of structural integrity is concerned. This self-protecting phenomenon, called *passivation,* is responsible for the near invulnerability to corrosion of many of our most useful metals and alloys including aluminum in airplanes, chrome-plated-steel auto trim, stainless steel cookware, and titanium chemical-plant piping. To be effective, the passive film must possess a number of attributes:

1. It must form on and adhere to metal surface.
2. It must be chemically stable in the surrounding environment.
3. It must form without cracks, pores, or pinholes.
4. It must provide a good barrier to the outward migration of metal ions and the inward migration of oxygen.
5. It must be relatively hard and abrasion resistant.
6. It must be able to repair any damage that occurs.

The self-repair feature is very important and stems directly from the electrochemical nature of most metal corrosion. If the passive film is ruptured by a scratch, the exposed metal immediately becomes an anode because it is much more reactive than the surrounding surface, which is still protected by the film and therefore acts as a cathode. Note, however, that the cathode reaction is slow because it is controlled by diffusion through the film. Nevertheless, the cathode area is orders of magnitude greater than that of the anode, so the overall cathode reaction (i.e., the rate of electron uptake) is sufficient to allow the anode reaction to proceed rapidly. In this way the scratch is quickly filled up with corrosion products (figure 15.5).

It is important to emphasize at this point that, whenever corrosion resistance depends on the presence of a passive film, the environment must be well oxygenated to maintain and repair the film. This requirement is usually, but not always, satisfied for orthopaedic implants in the physiological environment.

■ 15.5 IMPLANT ALLOYS

An important factor that must be considered when placing passivated alloys in the physiological environment is the presence of chloride ion. Chloride-containing solutions are, in general, much more aggressive

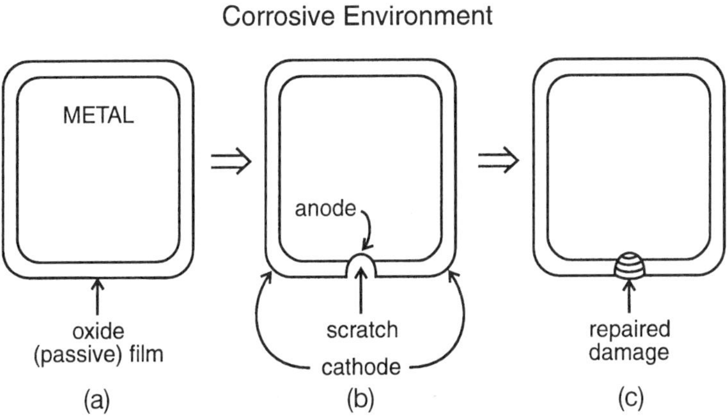

Figure 15.5. *(a)* A metal component protected from environmental attack by an oxide (passive) film. *(b)* Rupture of the film by a scratch, leading to creation of a small anodic region and a large, new, cathodic region. *(c)* Rapid repair of the scratch.

than those lacking this ion, and many alloys loose their passive resistance when this species is present. Two notable exceptions to this rule are titanium and chromium, and it is no accident that all standard orthopaedic implant alloys contain one or the other of these elements. Both titanium and chromium form very stable oxides with heats of formation respectively of -218 kcal/mole and -270 kcal/mole. Because they are harder than glass, they have good abrasion resistance, but the films formed under ambient conditions are only a few hundred atoms thick. For this reason, implant manufacturers expose their components to special passivating treatments to increase the thickness of the films. Even then the film thickness is less than 0.1 μm or about 1% of the diameter of a red blood cell.

The titanium alloy 6Al-4V is slightly less corrosion resistant than pure titanium. This slight compromise of corrosion resistance is accepted in order to take advantage of the greater strength of the alloy, which is needed for load-bearing orthopaedic implants. The situation with the iron-based alloy (stainless steel) and cobalt-based alloys is different. In both these cases, passivity depends on the addition of chromium as an alloying element. When chromium is present in sufficiently high concentrations, these alloys form complex oxide films that contain both chromium and the solvent metal, for example, ($M_x O_y \cdot Cr_2 O_3$).

As discussed in chapter 14, the cobalt-chromium-molybdenum (Co-Cr-Mo) alloys have complex microstructures that in some compositions include substantial amounts of metal carbides as a second phase. These microstructures, not withstanding these alloys, have compiled a record of outstanding corrosion resistance since their introduction as surgical implants more than 50 years ago.

The austenitic stainless steel alloys are also protected by a mixed-oxide film based on $Cr_2 O_3$. Iron-based alloys must contain a minimum of 12% chromium in order to develop a true passive film. In the 316 alloy, the chromium content is elevated to 17%–19%, and nickel is added in the amounts of 12%–14% to improve corrosion resistance further. These alloys have simple, single-phase microstructures, but the oxide films are not as stable as those formed on the titanium and cobalt-chromium-molybdenum (Co-Cr-Mo) alloys. The increased galvanic potential for 316 stainless steel under conditions where passivity has been lost is shown by the black bar in figure 15.3. Because of this slightly lower corrosion resistance and the lower strength of austenitic stainless steels, these alloys are largely reserved for implant applications where their high ductility permits intraoperative bending and shaping. Typical applications include wire sutures, cerclage wires, fracture-fixation plates, and certain scoliosis-correction instrumentation, such as the Cotrel-Dubousset system.

■ 15.6 CREVICE CORROSION

A crevice is created whenever two components are held in close contact. Orthopaedic examples include a screw and fixation-plate combination and the ball and neck of a modular hip prosthesis. Crevices are typically a tenth of a millimeter or less, which is enough space for the environment (solution) to invade the crevice but not enough to maintain the nominal composition of the solution by convection and agitation. In this circumstance, the dissolved oxygen trapped in the crevice will eventually be consumed by the reduction reaction. This does not mean that the anodic reaction (metal ionization) is also stopped. Rather, further release of metal ions causes both chloride and hydrogen ions to migrate into the crevice, leading to a local environment that is notably low in oxygen but has an elevated chloride content and lowered pH. This altered local environment is much more corrosive than the ambient physiological fluid and can lead to detectable attack on metals that lose their passivity easily. Unfortunately, austenitic stainless steels fall in this category, and detectable corrosion can almost always be found in screw/plate fixation systems that have been in place for any extended period of time. Both the titanium alloy and the cobalt-chromium-molybdenum (Co-Cr-Mo) alloys are more resistant to crevice corrosion than stainless steel, and it is in this sense that these alloys are said to have superior corrosion resistance. Unfortunately, even the titanium and cobalt-based alloys show crevice-corrosion effects in modular hip systems, and methods are under development to cope with this potentially serious problem. In particular, it is now strongly recommended that cobalt-chromium-molybdenum (Co-Cr-Mo) balls not be used with Ti 6Al-4V stems because even the small difference in the galvanic potential between these two alloy systems is enough to set up a corrosion cell that enhances crevice corrosion. This, of course, is precisely the predicament that Dr. Curmudgeon unknowingly stepped into when his scrub nurse gave him a cobalt-chromium-molybdenum (Co-Cr-Mo) head to place on a Ti 6Al/4V stem. We will shortly consider the possible problems that might grow out of this unfortunate choice. In general, it is a good idea always to avoid the coupling of dissimilar metals, especially if one of them is stainless steel.

■ 15.7 FRETTING CORROSION

Fretting refers to the rubbing that occurs across a mechanical joint, such as a screw and plate, when an intermittent load is applied. During fretting, the protective film is worn away even if the relative motion is microscopic in extent. This loss of the passive film in turn abets the crevice-corrosion process. Fretting is a particular problem for titanium components because titanium has a severe tendency to gall, or cold weld, to itself in rubbing situations. Fretting is well documented in modular hip systems as well as in screw/plate combinations.

■ 15.8 COLD WORK

When the surface of a metal specimen is scratched or dented, a small region of material is displaced to the sides of the defect. This material, although small in amount, undergoes considerable plastic deformation and as a result becomes anodic to the rest of the sample. For this reason, it is a good idea to avoid rough handling of implants, which always have surfaces that the manufacturer has carefully prepared to optimize corrosion resistance. Local plastic deformation is also likely to occur on the mating surfaces of multicomponent implants when they are assembled. For example, when a screw is seated against the screw hole in a plate, a thin layer of cold-worked metal is created where the two parts rub against each other during "setting" of the screw. This then becomes another factor contributing to crevice corrosion.

■ 15.9 PITTING CORROSION

Most metals that are protected from corrosion by a passive oxide film are subject to localized breakdown of the film and rapid local corrosion (i.e., pitting) when exposed to certain specific environments. As with so many other types of corrosion, this phenomenon is accentuated by the presence of chloride ion. The details of the pitting mechanism are complex and not yet fully understood and are not discussed here. It should be noted, however, that austenitic stainless steels are more prone to pitting in the physiological environment than the other implant alloys. However, the addition of small amounts of molybdenum (2%–4%) to austenitic stainless steels improves their resistance to pitting attack. For this reason, this alloy, designated 316 stainless steel, has become the standard for virtually all "stainless" orthopaedic implants.

■ 15.10 SENSITIZATION

Typically, austenitic stainless steels contain as much as 0.08% by weight of carbon. This seemingly small amount can have a vast effect on corrosion resistance, however, because carbon has a great propensity to form intermetallic compounds with chromium. Under certain processing conditions, chromium and carbon diffuse to the grain boundaries of austenitic stainless steels and precipitate as a chromium carbide (e.g., $Cr_{23}C_6$). In certain temperature ranges, the driving force (i.e., energy decrease) for the formation of this precipitate is so great that it proceeds rapidly until the chromium in rigorous adjacent-to-the-grain boundaries is depleted. This condition is known as sensitization (figure 15.6). When the local chromium content falls below 11% or 12%, the alloy reverts to its nonstainless condition, and a severe galvanic reaction occurs between the chromium-depleted zone and the rest of the grain. This leads to rapid attack along the grain boundaries and eventual failure of the component. Sensitization can be avoided if the carbon content is held to low enough levels. Whenever a batch of 316 stainless steel is produced with a carbon content below 0.03%, it is designated as 316L (the L stands for low carbon). As production-process controls improved, it became possible to produce these steels with even lower carbon contents. Batches with carbon contents less than 0.015% are now available and are designated as 316 ELC, for extra low carbon. As one might expect, a premium is charged for the L and ELC grades. Nonetheless, these grades are specified for all 316 stainless steel implants at the present time.

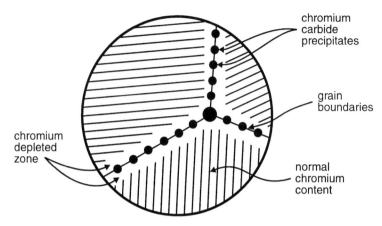

Figure 15.6. Grain boundaries with chromium carbide precipitates in an austenitic stainless steel. Regions adjacent to the grain boundaries are depleted in chromium due to formation of the precipitates. The chromium-lean regions then become anodic to the rest of the grain and are rapidly attacked in oxygenated saline solutions.

■ 15.11 ION RELEASE

With the exception of crevice corrosion, the corrosion experienced by orthopaedic implants is so slight that it cannot be detected by ordinary means such as microscopic examination or precise gravimetric (weighing) procedures. Measurements of corrosion currents using extremely sensitive electrical instruments and analysis of tissues using ultrasensitive chemical analysis procedures (such as atomic absorption spectroscopy and neutron activation analysis) have demonstrated that metal ions migrate through the oxide film and are released into the physiological environment in small amounts. The biological fate and clinical impact of these released ions is a subject of great complexity as suggested by table 15.3, which is a list of the primary factors involved in metal ion release. Treating this subject in depth is much beyond the scope of this primer, but some of the important concepts will be mentioned. Most of the metallic elements in orthopaedic alloys are naturally present in the body, some in fairly high concentrations and some as trace elements only. Many of the trace elements have indispensable physiological functions but become toxic at high concentrations. In evaluating the potential hazards due to metal-ion release, it is therefore

Table 15.3 Factors effecting the biological response to ions released by metal implants

Physicochemical
    Elemental species (toxicity)
    State of ionization
    Wear particle accumulation and phagocytosis
    Rate of ion release
    Peri-implant concentration
Biochemical
    Protein binding
    Transport from the implant site
    Excretion route and rate
    Accumulation in organs
Host reactions
    Encapsulation
    Inflammation
    Infection potentiation
    Immune system compromise
    Allergic response
    Tumor potentiation and induction
    Dose-response relationships for all of the above

crucial for clinicians and researchers to know what the peri-implant and systemic concentrations are and to compare these with the dose levels that produce toxicity and other undesirable effects. In general, proteins coat all implants, tending to isolate them from the physiological environment and to reduce the rate of ion release. Furthermore, binding of the metal ions by proteins is common and can have either beneficial or detrimental effects. Protein-bound metal ions may be transported away from the implant site by active processes, thus keeping the local concentration low. On the other hand, binding metal ions can alter the protein so that it is recognized as an antigen by the body, setting off an immune or allergic reaction. In this regard, both nickel and chromium ions have been shown to be able to provoke an allergic reaction in many patients, and this is probably a contributing factor in some chronic implant problems. A particular concern is chromium ion in the +6 valence state, which has been implicated as a tumor-potentiating, or tumor-inducing, agent.

Much research is needed in this area, and the young orthopaedist would be well advised to stay abreast of developments as she or he follows the profession in the years to come.

■ 15.12 CONCLUSION

Dr. Curmudgeon's unfortunate choice of a cobalt-chromium-molybdenum (Co-Cr-Mo) head to go with a Ti 6Al/4V stem is likely to lead to a crevice-corrosion situation that will be exacerbated by the dissimilar metals involved. Examination of corrosion products recovered from such crevices show clear evidence of nickel- and chromium-compound formation, which suggests that an allergic reaction—or worse—could be in this patient's future.

Q15: Clinical Question (Summary)

After placing a titanium shaft into the femoral canal one day, Dr. Curmedgeon was not aware that the scrub nurse had handed him a cobalt-chromium-alloy (Co-Cr) femoral head of the appropriate size. Is the difference in the two metals likely to cause any problems, and, if so, what sort of problems should we expect?

A15: Clinical Answer

As was stated in Section 15.12, Dr. Curmudgeon's unfortunate choice of a cobalt-chromium-molybdenum head to go with a Ti 6Al/4V stem is likely to lead to a crevice-corrosion situation that will be exacerbated by the dissimilar metals involved. Examination of corrosion products recovered from such crevices show clear evidence of nickel and chromium-compound formation, which suggests that an allergic reaction—or worse—could be in this patient's future.

Additional Reading

Fontana MG: *Corrosion Engineering.* McGraw-Hill, New York, 1986.

Lemons JE: Corrosion and biodegradation. In *Handbook of Biomaterials Evaluation,* AF von Recum, Ed. Macmillan, New York, p. 109, 1986.

Levine DL: *Metal Degradation in the Taper Connection of Modular Hip Prostheses.* Technical Monograph 97–2000–146. Zimmer, Warsaw, Ind., 1996.

Sharkness CM, Acosta SK, More RM, Hamburger S, Gross TP: Metallic orthopaedic implants and their possible association with cancer. *J Long Term Ef Med Implants* 3(3):237, 1993.

Syrett BC, Acharya A (Eds): *Corrosion and Degradation of Implant Materials.* ASTM STP 684. American Society for Testing and Materials, West Conshohocken, Pa., 1979.

Williams DF (Ed): *Fundamental Aspects of Biocompatibility,* vols. I and II. CRC Press, Boca Raton, Fla., 1981.

Urban RM, Joshua JJ, Gilbert JL, Rice SB, Jasty M, Bragdon CR, Galante JO: Characterization of Solid Particles of Corrosion Generated by Modular-Head Femoral Stems of Different Designs and Materials. In *Modularity of Orthopaedic Implants,* DE Marlowe, JE Parr, MB Mayor, Eds. ASTM STP 1301. Am Soc Testing and Mats, West Conshohocken, Pa., p. 33, 1997.

Williams DF, Williams RL: Degradative Effects of the Biological Environment on Metals and Ceramics. In *Biomaterials Science,* BD Ratner, AS Hoffman, FJ Schoen, JL Lemons, Eds. Academic Press, San Diego, p. 260, 1996.

16

Orthopaedic Polymers

CLINICAL SCENARIO: POLYETHYLENE WEAR IN TOTAL KNEE COMPONENTS

The Mainstream twins' friend Pearl had an arthritic knee that had been treated by implant arthroplasty, and she was doing very well indeed. She was able to do virtually anything she wished, but in recent months she had begun to have pain in the knee. Because the discomfort limited her walking ability, she made an appointment to see her surgeon, who told her she needed a revision operation. When the surgeon opened the knee, he found the femoral component intact but the plastic on the tibial side badly worn. These modern plastic components should last forever, should they not? What happened to this one?

Plastics (or polymers) are used in many different forms in orthopaedics. Two common orthopaedic polymers that we will discuss in some detail in this chapter are polyethylene and polymethyl methacrylate (or bone cement).

■ 16.1 BASIC CHARACTERISTICS OF POLYMERS

Polymers are large molecules built up by the repetition of small, simple chemical units. In fact, the word *polymer* means many units, as derived from the terms *poly* (which means *many*) and *mer* (which means *unit*). One unit of the repeating pattern of a polymer is then a monomer.

Human-made polymers were first introduced in the 1930s; development of new polymers continues to the present day. Some important polymers used in medicine, their chemical formulas, and the monomer from which they are derived are given in table 16.1.

The microstructure of polymers is usually in the form of chains that have strong covalent bonding of the chain backbone. The bonds along the chain backbone are usually carbon-to-carbon (C-C) covalent bonds; however, there are many polymers with different backbone compositions. Polymers are generally formed by either addition polymerization or condensation polymerization.

16.1.1 Addition Polymerization

In addition polymerization, the starting mer contains a double bond (for example, ethylene; when a free radical, $R\cdot$, is added, it reacts with a mer to create an unsatisfied bond (figure 16.1).

This newly created open bond then reacts with another mer, and the molecule grows. If only a small amount of free radical is added (only a few chains are started), and few contaminants are present (that can terminate the chains), then the chains can grow to great length.

In the example just given, the starting mer was *ethylene,* so the resulting polymer is *polyethylene* (the polymer is always named for the starting mer). The polyethylene used for acetabular cups in total hip arthroplasty has a molecular weight of $3-6 \times 10^6$g/mol.

Free radicals are molecules that can dissociate readily and, in the dissociated form, are highly reactive. A molecule of this type that is used in a number of addition polymerization reactions is benzoyl peroxide (see figure 16.2).

The O–O bond in benzoyl peroxide may rupture spontaneously or may be broken by the input of a small amount of energy in the form of heat, light, or the enthalpy released by an adjacent (activator) reaction.

16.1.2 Condensation Polymerization

In condensation polymerization, the chemical reaction of mers with symmetrical end (functional) groups is involved rather than the rearrangement of double bonds. In condensation polymerization, a small molecule (e.g., water [H_2O] or carbon dioxide [CO_2]) is often released (or "condensed out") as a reaction by-product. This, of course, is where

Table 16.1 Chemical Formulas of some common biomedical polymers

Polymer	Repeating unit	Monomer
Polyethylene (PE)	$-\overset{\text{H}}{\underset{\text{H}}{\text{C}}}-\left[\overset{\text{H}}{\underset{\text{H}}{\text{C}}}-\overset{\text{H}}{\underset{\text{H}}{\text{C}}}\right]-\overset{\text{H}}{\underset{\text{H}}{\text{C}}}-$	$\overset{\text{H}}{\underset{\text{H}}{\text{C}}}=\overset{\text{H}}{\underset{\text{H}}{\text{C}}}$
Polyvinyl chloride (PVC)	$-CH_2-\overset{\text{H}}{\underset{\text{Cl}}{\text{C}}}-\left[CH_2-\overset{\text{H}}{\underset{\text{Cl}}{\text{C}}}\right]-CH_2-\overset{\text{H}}{\underset{\text{Cl}}{\text{C}}}-$	$\overset{\text{H}}{\underset{\text{H}}{\text{C}}}=\overset{\text{H}}{\underset{\text{Cl}}{\text{C}}}$
Polyvinyl alcohol (PVA)	$-CH_2-\overset{\text{H}}{\underset{\text{OH}}{\text{C}}}-\left[CH_2-\overset{\text{H}}{\underset{\text{OH}}{\text{C}}}\right]-CH_2-\overset{\text{H}}{\underset{\text{OH}}{\text{C}}}-$	$\overset{\text{H}}{\underset{\text{H}}{\text{C}}}=\overset{\text{H}}{\underset{\text{OH}}{\text{C}}}$
Polymethyl metha-crylate (PMMA)	$-CH_2-\underset{\underset{\text{O}}{\overset{\text{C=O}}{\mid}}{\overset{\text{CH}_3}{\text{C}}}...-CH_2-\text{C}...$ (with CH_3 top, $C=O$, O, CH_3)	$\overset{\text{H}}{\underset{\text{H}}{\text{C}}}=\overset{\text{CH}_3}{\underset{\substack{\text{C=O}\\\mid\\\text{O}\\\mid\\\text{CH}_3}}{\text{C}}}$
Polytetrafluoroethy-lene (PTFE or Teflon*)	$-\overset{\text{F}}{\underset{\text{F}}{\text{C}}}-\overset{\text{F}}{\underset{\text{F}}{\text{C}}}-\left[\overset{\text{F}}{\underset{\text{F}}{\text{C}}}-\overset{\text{F}}{\underset{\text{F}}{\text{C}}}\right]-\overset{\text{F}}{\underset{\text{F}}{\text{C}}}-\overset{\text{F}}{\underset{\text{F}}{\text{C}}}-$	$\overset{\text{F}}{\underset{\text{F}}{\text{C}}}=\overset{\text{F}}{\underset{\text{F}}{\text{C}}}$
Polyester (Example: PET or Poly(ethyleneter-ephthalate))	$\left[-O-C_2H_4-O-\overset{\overset{\text{O}}{\|\|}}{\text{C}}-C_6H_4-\overset{\overset{}{}}{\underset{\|\|}{\text{C}}}\underset{\text{O}}{}-\right]$	
Polyurethanes* (*R_1 & R_2 are aliphatic,cycloali-phatic, aromatic)	$\left[-R_1-\overset{\text{H}}{\text{N}}-\overset{\overset{\text{O}}{\|\|}}{\text{C}}-O-R_2O-\right]$	

*Registered trademark of E. I. du Pont de Nemours & Co.

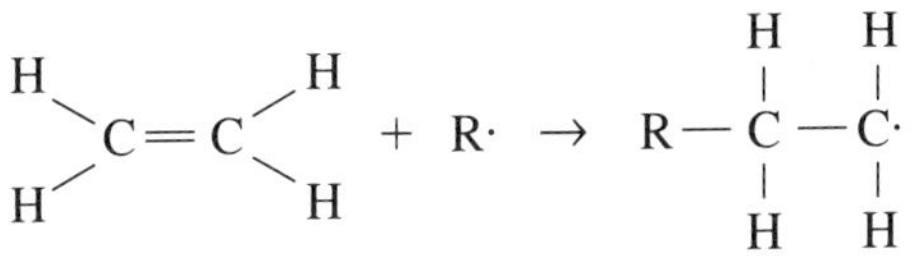

$$
\underset{H}{\overset{H}{\diagdown}} C = C \underset{H}{\overset{H}{\diagup}} \quad + \quad R \cdot \quad \rightarrow \quad R - \overset{\displaystyle H}{\underset{\displaystyle H}{\overset{|}{\underset{|}{C}}}} - \overset{\displaystyle H}{\underset{\displaystyle H}{\overset{|}{\underset{|}{C}}}} \cdot
$$

Figure 16.1. Representation of addition of a free radical to form a reacting chain in addition polymerization.

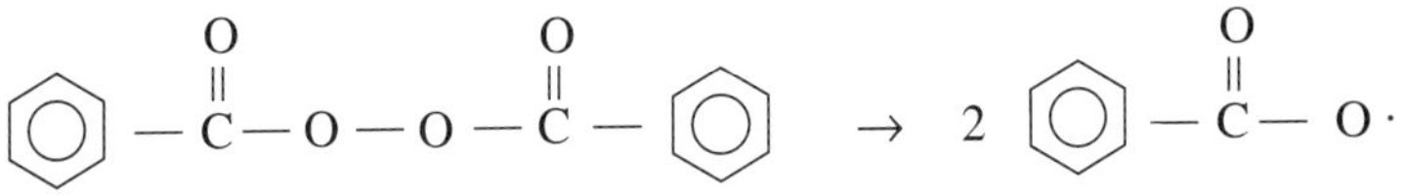

$$
\bigcirc - \overset{O}{\overset{||}{C}} - O - O - \overset{O}{\overset{||}{C}} - \bigcirc \quad \rightarrow \quad 2 \ \bigcirc - \overset{O}{\overset{||}{C}} - O \cdot
$$

Figure 16.2. The breaking of benzoyl peroxide to form reactive free radicals.

this particular method of polymerization gets its name. Other reactions that release no products at all can still produce condensation polymers. The important factor is the chemical reaction of symmetrical end groups. Examples of polymers made by condensation polymerization are polyethylene terephthalate (PET) and polyurethane.

■ 16.2 STRUCTURAL FORMULAS OF POLYMERS

Formulas that indicate the structure of a polymer usually consist of the formula for the starting mer enclosed in brackets with the average molecular weight indicated by a subscript. For example, polyethylene is written as shown in figure 16.3, where a typical n would be 5×10^6.

If the starting mer, $C = C-C$ (propylene), is used instead of ethylene, the resulting polymerization is as shown in figure 16.4a, and the polymer is as shown in figure 16.4b.

In other words, polypropylene and polyethylene differ from each other in that polypropylene has a methyl group attached to every other

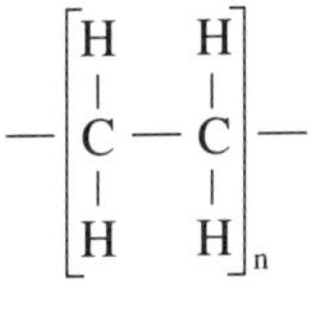

$$
- \left[\overset{\displaystyle H}{\underset{\displaystyle H}{\overset{|}{\underset{|}{C}}}} - \overset{\displaystyle H}{\underset{\displaystyle H}{\overset{|}{\underset{|}{C}}}} \right]_n -
$$

Figure 16.3. The structural formula for polyethylene.

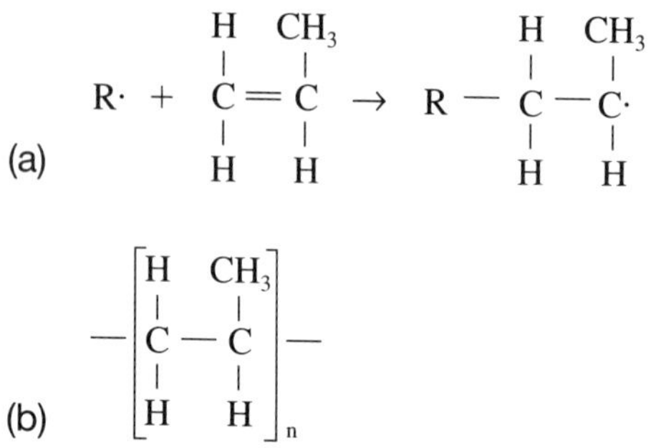

$$\text{R·} \; + \; \underset{\underset{\text{H}}{|}}{\overset{\overset{\text{H}}{|}}{\text{C}}} = \underset{\underset{\text{H}}{|}}{\overset{\overset{\text{CH}_3}{|}}{\text{C}}} \; \rightarrow \; \text{R} - \underset{\underset{\text{H}}{|}}{\overset{\overset{\text{H}}{|}}{\text{C}}} - \underset{\underset{\text{H}}{|}}{\overset{\overset{\text{CH}_3}{|}}{\text{C·}}}$$

(a)

$$- \left[\underset{\underset{\text{H}}{|}}{\overset{\overset{\text{H}}{|}}{\text{C}}} - \underset{\underset{\text{H}}{|}}{\overset{\overset{\text{CH}_3}{|}}{\text{C}}} \right]_n -$$

(b)

Figure 16.4. A simple representation of the addition polymerization process for (a) polypropylene and (b) the resulting structural formula.

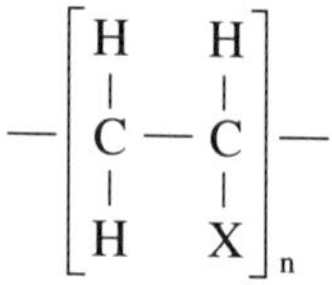

$$- \left[\underset{\underset{\text{H}}{|}}{\overset{\overset{\text{H}}{|}}{\text{C}}} - \underset{\underset{\text{X}}{|}}{\overset{\overset{\text{H}}{|}}{\text{C}}} \right]_n -$$

Figure 16.5. The structural formula for a vinyl. Replacing the X side group forms different types of polymers that are generically grouped as vinyls.

C in the backbone molecule. This general arrangement is characteristic of a large family of polymers called vinyls, as shown in figure 16.5, where the X position may be occupied by any atom or functional group (see table 16.1). For an example, see figure 16.6.

A similar polymer important in medicine is polytetrafluoroethylene (Teflon). It should be obvious that the structural formula is as shown in figure 16.7.

■ 16.3 STRENGTH OF POLYMERS

The addition and condensation polymers considered up to this point consist of chains that have little or no branching or cross-linking to neighboring chains. Such simple chain polymers are called linear polymers. Linear polymers derive their strength (in the bulk) from the entanglement of the chains. Weak bonding forces (e.g., Van der Waals

Table 16.2 Vinyl type polymers based on polyethylene where different functional groups are substituted for one hydrogen atom at the x-position

X	Polymer
–H	Polyethylene
–CH3	Polypropylene
–Cl	Polyvinyl chloride
–OH	Polyvinyl alcohol
–ethyl	Polybutylene
–phenyl	Polystyrene

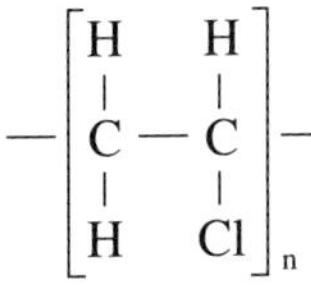

$$-\begin{bmatrix} \begin{array}{cc} H & H \\ | & | \\ C & - C \\ | & | \\ H & Cl \end{array} \end{bmatrix}_n-$$

Figure 16.6. The structural formula for polyvinyl chloride.

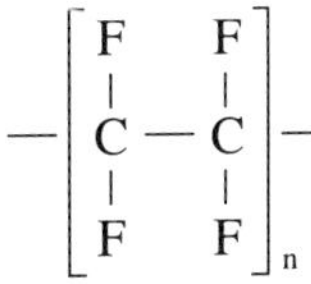

$$-\begin{bmatrix} \begin{array}{cc} F & F \\ | & | \\ C & - C \\ | & | \\ F & F \end{array} \end{bmatrix}_n-$$

Figure 16.7. The structural formula for polytetrafluoroethylene (Teflon).

bonds) prevent one chain from slipping past another. Therefore, the more points of contact across which these weak bonds can interact, the stronger the bulk polymer will be. As a practical matter, anything that increases the number of bonding sites will increase the strength of the polymer.

16.3.1 Molecular Weight

By far the most important single factor in increasing strength is the average molecular weight (i.e., chain length) of the polymer. As the chain length increases, the entanglement increases, as does the number of Van der Waals–type bonds per chain. A typical example of the effect of molecular weight on the strength of the polymer is shown for polyethylene in figure 16.8. The relationship between molecular weight and general mechanical properties is neither linear nor necessarily the same for each polymer. At the monomer level, ethylene is a gas. As the molecular weight is increased, the polyethylene polymer turns first into a liquid, then a soft wax, and finally a useful structural material.

In general, the following occur as molecular weight *increases:*

- Tensile strength *increases*
- Shear strength *increases*
- Toughness *increases*
- Softening temperature *increases*
- Impact resistance *increases*
- Resistance to environmental attack *increases*
- Melt fluidity *decreases*
- Fabricability *decreases*

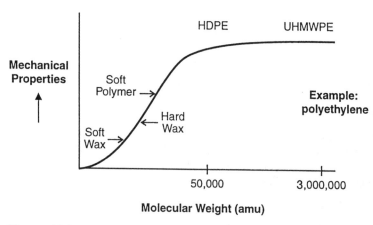

Figure 16.8. The properties of a polymer depend on its molecular weight. In this simple example for polyethylene, increasing the molecular weight generally increases its mechanical properties, such as strength and wear resistance.

- Coefficient of friction *decreases*
- Solubility *decreases*

For polyethylene, there is not much difference in mechanical properties of material between the molecular weights of 50,000 amu and 2,000,000 amu. Two different mechanisms of strengthening of the polymer occur in these two types of polyethylene. In the 50,000-amu material, crystallinity is a strengthening mechanism; in the 2,000,000-amu material, chain entanglement is more important. The difference in these two mechanisms is discussed in the next section.

16.3.2 Crystallinity

In chapter 13, a crystal was defined as a substance whose constituent atoms or molecules are arranged in an orderly pattern that repeats over long distances in three dimensions. Materials that exhibit no such long-range order are called amorphous. Glass is an example. As one might anticipate, most linear polymers are amorphous because of the random entanglement of the molecules. In some cases, slow cooling from the melt can facilitate the arrangement of the polymer molecules in parallel arrays that satisfy all the requirements of a crystal. A two-dimensional example is given in figure 16.9.

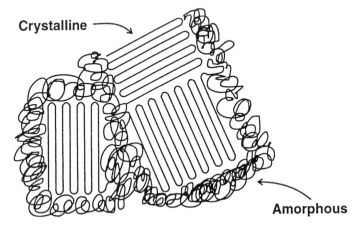

Figure 16.9. High-density polyethylene (and some other linear polymers) can be highly crystalline. Crystallinity is achieved by the folding of chains. Amorphous (or nonordered) regions form between crystalline regions.

Unlike metal and ceramic materials, where every atom is positioned in the crystal, polymers are usually partly crystalline and partly amorphous. The percent crystallinity is usually given for well-characterized polymers. Polymers are often 100% amorphous but seldom attain more than 90% crystallinity.

Crystallinity contributes to strength because the orderly arrangement of the chains permits them to come into close approximation at a greater number of points than is possible in a tangled amorphous structure. Because the weak interchain bonds work only at points of close approximation of the chains, there are more active bonding sites and hence a greater overall strength as the percent crystallinity increases. Interestingly, the chains are more tightly packed in a crystal; thus the density of the polymer increases slightly as the percent crystallinity increases.

Finally, the ability to form crystalline structures depends on the molecular weight of the polymer. For extremely long chains (high molecular weight), the chains entangled in the melt are not readily reorganized into the crystal arrangement. Thus one strengthening mechanism—high molecular weight—is at odds with another, crystallinity. It is hard to take advantage of both mechanisms in the same polymer.

An important example of this is polyethylene. This polymer is produced in several forms: One is highly crystalline with a moderately high molecular weight (~50,000 amu), and another is an ultrahigh molecular weight material (3,000,000 amu) with a completely amorphous structure. Some properties for these two forms of polyethylene are listed in table 16.3. The highly crystalline material also has a higher density and is called high-density polyethylene (HDPE), whereas the ultrahigh molecular weight material is designated UHMWPE. Why is

Table 16.3 Properties of HD and UHMW polyethylene

	HDPE	UHMWPE
Mol. wt. (g/mol)	$1–2 \times 10^5$	$3–6 \times 10^6$
Density (g/cm^3)	0.94–0.96	0.93–0.94
Crystallinity (%)	70–90	
Tensile strength (MPa)	23–40	27–34

the density of HDPE higher than for UHMWPE? More information on these materials will be presented in Section 16.4.2.

16.3.3 Temperature

When linear polymers are heated, the added thermal energy causes the chains to wiggle and vibrate. This activity assists chains in slipping past each other. On the macroscopic level, the bulk polymer becomes soft and eventually melts. If allowed to cool, the polymer will regain its room-temperature strength. In addition, such melting and rehardening can be repeated numerous times. Such polymers are called *thermopolymers,* or *thermoplastics.* The ability to melt and then regain strength is a great asset in forming thermopolymers into desired shapes. Early thermopolymers were called plastics because of this easy formability, but this term is no longer used in the technical/scientific literature.

Polymers that do not melt but only soften slightly and then decompose at higher temperatures are referred to as thermoset polymers. Rubber, epoxies, and other cross-linked polymers (polymers that have covalent bonding between individual chains) are thermoset polymers. They do not melt because the energy to overcome the covalent bonds (so that the segments can flow past each other) is equal to the energy needed to break the chains apart. Have you ever wondered why squealing tires on a quick start is called "burning rubber" and not "melting rubber"? Now you know!

16.3.4 Additives

Many additives are incorporated into polymers for a variety of reasons, both intentional and unavoidable. Most of these additives affect the strength and other characteristics of the base polymer.

PLASTICIZERS. Many polymers, especially those intended for high-volume, high-rate commercial fabrication, are supplied with additives of small, low molecular weight organic molecules called plasticizers. They separate the molecular chains of the polymer, thus reducing its strength, especially at moderately elevated temperatures. Although this may detract from service performance to some degree, it greatly facilitates formation at high temperatures and thus reduces costs.

Have you ever wondered why—when they started out so supple—plastic dashboards and plastic parts of seats in old cars crack? One reason is that the plasticizer molecules are not chemically bound to the polymer molecules. As a result, they can be leached out of the polymer, and, because they are small, chemically active moieties, they are likely to be toxic. For this reason, manufacturers avoid using polymers with plasticizers for surgical implants. For many important commercial polymers, it is essentially impossible to obtain shipments with no plasticizing additions, and, as a result, these materials have not found favor as implants. Polymers that are free or nearly free of plasticizers are more costly to produce.

An important but unintended example of plasticization is the absorption of water or lipids by polymer implants. This can lead to softening of the implant in some cases and embrittlement in others. The failure of early silicone rubber finger joint prostheses may have been accelerated by lipid-absorption embrittlement.

OTHER ADDITIVES.   Other additives produce coloration, increase ultraviolet damage resistance and oxidation resistance, and initiate or enhance polymerization. All these additives are potentially leachable and therefore contra-indicated for surgical implants unless tested and found nontoxic and nondetrimental to mechanical properties (for example, methylene blue in bone cement).

16.3.5 Branching and Cross-Linking

An additional and very effective method of strengthening polymers is to produce chains that are branched or cross-linked. Branched chains are basically variants of linear structures. The branching improves strength by enhancing entanglement but eliminates crystallization by preventing the regular close arrangement of the chains that is required.

Cross-linked polymers are qualitatively different from linear polymers if the cross-linking is at all extensive. A schematic of a cross-linked polymer is shown in figure 16.10. The reason for this is that the interchain bonds that prevent the molecules from slipping are strong covalent bonds. Thus modest heating does not produce softening, and shapes cannot be produced in this way. The cross-linking is itself a kind of polymerization reaction and must be induced to occur simultaneously with the molding or shaping of the base resin.

For thermoset polymers, the concept of molecular weight loses most of its meaning because all the original molecules are covalently linked to their neighbors. It is tempting to think of the whole object as being composed of a single molecule with many interconnections that form a

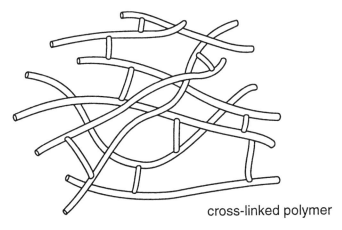

cross-linked polymer

Figure 16.10. Cross-linked polymers have covalent bonds between chain lengths. *Source:* Budinski K: *Engineering Materials, Properties and Selection,* 2d ed. Prentice-Hall, Reston, VA, 1983, p. 47, figure 3.7.

three-dimensional network. Thermoset polymers are generally stronger and stiffer than thermopolymers. The best of the modern thermopolymers are beginning to compete successfully with the thermosets, however. Epoxies are the most common and most important thermoset polymers. Because of their toxicity, they are not used for surgical implants but are widely used in ancillary medical equipment and devices, especially as adhesives.

16.3.6 Fillers

Many polymers are strengthened, and their abrasion resistance is particularly improved by mixing in fine particles of a hard substance. Examples include graphite (lampblack) in latex rubber (for tires), glass particles in epoxy, and barium sulfate ($BaSO_4$, an X-ray opacifier) in bone cement. In the last example, the barium sulfate particles do not improve the strength of the bone cement because no attempt has been made to bond the particles to the matrix polymer. Fillers are effective strengtheners only if they are strongly bonded to the matrix polymer.

Many different polymers are used in the biomedical industry. The trade names used for these polymers vary from company to company and can represent differences in the way the polymer is formed (e.g., bulk, sheet, or fibers), the molecular weight, and so on. Several biomedical plastics and some of their proprietary names are listed in table 16.4.

■ 16.4 IMPORTANT ORTHOPAEDIC POLYMERS: BONE CEMENT AND POLYETHYLENE

16.4.1 Bone Cement

Bone cement is a grouting medium used to fix a prosthesis in place. The most common type of bone cement is PMMA bone cement, where PMMA is short for polymethyl methacrylate, an acrylic polymer that has the same basic chemical composition as Plexiglas.

PMMA was first discovered as a biocompatible material when Plexiglas shards from airplane windshields embedded in the eyes of pilots did not cause a reaction by the body. Early use of PMMA in medicine was as a denture material and a substance to repair skull defects. PMMA bone cement was first popularized in the early 1960s by an English orthopaedic surgeon, Sir John Charnley. Although not the first to use PMMA as a bone cement, Sir John did develop the cementing method upon which modern cement techniques are based. A dental materials scientist named Dr. Dennis Smith introduced Sir John to PMMA dental cement. The two collaborated on developing a PMMA bone cement that was radioopaque and could be polymerized in vivo. With some minor revisions, the cement formulation they developed is still used in most bone cements on the market today.

> Did you know that for several years in the early 1960s, patients who had cemented total hip replacements had the operation done with pink bone cement? This was not to facilitate locating the cement in revision surgery. The cement was pink because it was originally intended to be used in making dentures!

Table 16.4 The proprietary names of some common biomedical plastics

Chemical name	Proprietary name
Polyethylene	Polythene
	Alkathene
	Carlona
	Marlex
	Alathon
	Hylamer
Polypropylene	Propathene
Polytetrafluoroethylene (PTFE)	Teflon
	Fluon
Polymethyl methacrylate (PMMA)	Acrylic
	Diakon
	Lucite
	Oroglas
	Perspex
	Plexiglas
Polyacetal (polyformaldehyde, polyoxymethylene)	Delrin
Polyacrylonitrile	Orlon
	Courtelle
Polyethylene terephthalate	Dacron (fiber)
	Mylar (film)
Polyurethane	Estane
	Lycra
	Polyfoam
Polyvinylalcohol (formalinized)	Ivalon
	Formvar
Polydimethyl siloxane (silicon rubber)	Silastic
Regenerated cellulose	Cellophane
Viscose rayon	Surgicel
Polyhydroxyethyl methacrylate	Hydron

The most common commercial bone cements today are supplied as a 20-ml vial of liquid (monomer) and a 40-g bag of powder (spheres of PMMA). Sterilization methods of the components are membrane filtration for the liquid and gamma radiation for the powder.

Following is the chemical composition of the liquid:

- MMA monomer
    - ≈ 97.5 v/o
- Toluidine
    - ≈ 2.5 v/o
    - promotes cold curing
    - also known as the accelerator
- Hydroquinone
    - ≈ 75 ppm
    - inhibits unwanted early polymerization
    - also called the inhibitor

Following is the chemical composition of the powder:

- Spherical particles of PMMA or PMMA copolymer
    - ≈ 88 w/o
    - particle size ranges from 30 to 150 μm in diameter
- Barium sulfate
    - ≈ 10 w/o
    - radiopacifier
- benzoyl peroxide
    - ≈ 2 w/o
    - initiator

16.4.1.1 Chemical Reaction of PMMA Bone Cement

PMMA bone cement is polymerized through addition polymerization in an exothermic reaction. To start the polymerization process, the liquid and powder are mixed together. The polymerization process occurs in three basic stages: initiation, propagation, and termination. There are four distinct consistency stages during the mixing of PMMA bone cement; the duration of each stage and the consistency of the cement during each stage are important for the use of bone cement in surgery. There are four macroscopic stages of mixing and setting:

1. Sandy stage (the monomer and powder look like they are not mixing together at all)

2. Stringy (the mixture is fluidlike and runny)

3. Doughy (the mixture is a soft mass and eventually does not stick to gloves upon handling)

4. Rigid mass (the cement becomes hard and solid and gets warm from the exothermic polymerization reaction)

The duration of each these consistency stages is important for use of the bone cement in surgery. The working time of bone cement was defined in early applied research as the time between the onset of the dough stage and the halfway point to maximum temperature (figure 16.11). The working time, quality of cement, and maximum temperature the cement reaches are controlled by a number of variables. These variables include ambient temperature, powder-to-liquid ratio, time of placement into the patient, and size, thickness, and mass of cement. Each factor is discussed next.

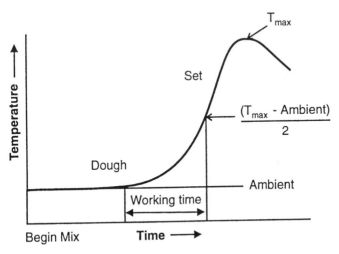

Figure 16.11. The temperature and viscosity of bone cement change with time as the cement is mixed and polymerizes. The working time has been defined as the time to reach the halfway point to the final change in temperature during polymerization. *Source:* Meyer PR, Lautenschlager EP, Moore BK: On the setting properties of acrylic bone cement. *J Bone Joint Surg* 55A(1):149–156, 1973, p. 150, figure 1.

16.4.1.2 Variables in Bone-Cement Setting

AMBIENT TEMPERATURE. As the ambient temperature increases, the working time decreases. Because the bone cement is affected by both global room and local temperature changes, one must look at both when considering ambient temperature. Common causes for shift in ambient temperature include the following:

- Variable air conditioners
- Holding the material in warm hands
- Mixing near warm lights
- Mixing in a warm bowl just removed from the sterilizer
- Holding the bowl in which the cement is mixed in one's warm hands.

➤ ⇑ ambient temperature → ⇓ working time

POWDER-TO-LIQUID RATIO. At first glance, it may seem like a good idea to add more monomer to the bone-cement mixture to make it less viscous. However, altering the powder-to-liquid ratio (P/L ratio) changes more than just the viscosity of the mix. Increasing the amount of liquid monomer [from the standard 2:1 P/L ratio (milligrams to milliliters)] decreases the P/L ratio. Decreasing the P/L ratio from the standard results in an increase in exothermic temperature in the cement and in setting time. Studies have also shown that the standard 2:1 P/L ratio minimizes the monomer loss from the bone cement. Either increasing or decreasing the P/L ratio increases the amount of monomer loss.

➤ ⇑ amount of liquid → ⇓ P/L ratio

➤ ⇓ P/L ratio → ⇑ heat released
⇑ setting time

➤ ⇕ P/L ratio → ⇑ monomer loss

TIME OF PLACEMENT INTO THE PATIENT. Studies show that the monomer loss in bone cement is greatest after cement starts to set.

Therefore, waiting to apply cement right up to the time of setting to reduce monomer loss is not justified. However, polymerizing bone cement is pseudoplastic before it sets, which means that its apparent viscosity decreases with higher flow rates (pressurization). Even though the cement may seem very thick, when injected under pressure, it will flow.

SIZE, THICKNESS, AND MASS OF CEMENT.   As stated previously, the polymerization of bone cement is an exothermic reaction. The total heat released during this exothermic reaction is fixed by the amount of reacting monomer. If the amount of monomer is increased, the amount of released heat increases. The temperature achieved in the cement depends on the rate of heat output and the surface area over which the heat is dissipated. For example, for a given mass of polymerizing standard bone cement, a ball of cement (small surface-to-volume ratio) will achieve a much higher temperature than will a flat sheet (large surface-to-volume ratio). Studies show that a sheet of bone cement that is 1.0 cm thick and prepared without heat sinks present can actually reach temperatures of 100°C and boil the monomer. The clinical implications of this fact are clear: In total hip replacement, for example, the thickness of the cement mantle should be uniform and approximately 3–4 mm. If a prosthesis is offset so that part of the mantle is thick and the opposite side thin, the thin part is under higher than normal stress, and the thick part may cause tissue necrosis from the high temperatures generated.

16.4.1.3 Advances in Bone-Cement Technology

At present, nearly half of the clinical failures of cemented prostheses can be attributed either directly or indirectly to failure of the bone cement. Fatigue testing of bone cement shows the endurance limit of the cement to be less than the maximum stresses imposed in everyday activity. Extensive mechanical fatigue failure of the cement can cause implant loosening and pain. More often, though, the cement failure contributes indirectly to implant failure by accelerating third-body wear of the polyethylene. Therefore, a new bone cement that is able to withstand higher repetitive stresses before failure would be beneficial.

Researchers are currently working on this problem from several different angles. New chemical formulations of bone cement (other than the plain PMMA) that are tougher and have higher endurance limits are being developed and tested. An obstacle to clinical use of these cements may be the cost of FDA approval of the new material.

Composite reinforcement is another approach to toughening of bone cement. Unlike aerospace composites, composite bone cement must be able to be mixed intraoperatively; therefore, the use of long fibers and high-volume additions of fibers is prohibited. At present, several groups of researchers are developing techniques for adding small amounts of fibers to the bone cement.

16.4.2 Polyethylene

Currently, the bearing material of choice for use in orthopaedic total joint replacements is ultrahigh molecular weight polyethylene (UHMWPE). UHMWPE is a thermoplastic polymer that is biologically inert in bulk. UHMWPE is commonly used in industrial applications that require sliding wear resistance. In fact, the use of UHMWPE in medical applications is minuscule in comparison to industrial use. It was first used commercially in 1955, first used in hip prosthesis in 1963, and first used in knee prostheses in early 1970s.

By definition, UHMWPE has a molecular weight of at least 3,000,000 amu ($n \approx 10^5$), hence the term *ultrahigh* MWPE (most thermoplastic polymers have molecular weights between 10,000 and 1,000,000 amu). UHMWPE has a melting temperature between 135 and 138°C and a softening temperature of 70–80°C. For this reason, UHMWPE cannot be autoclaved; sterilization methods must use chemicals or irradiation. Details of the effects of sterilization on UHMWPE are discussed later in this chapter.

16.4.2.1 Processing and Fabrication of UHMWPE

UHMWPE is fabricated into parts by sintering (or moderate-temperature bonding) of virgin UHMWPE powder. Sintering of the powder is done because, at temperatures exceeding the melting point, UHMWPE molecules will cross-link in the presence of oxygen (O_2) and the resin becomes rubbery but will not flow. This is why the UHMWPE powder will flow during sintering, but the fabricated form is hard to reshape.

The most prevalent modes of processing UHMWPE are ram extrusion, compression molding, and direct-compression forming. The goal in each method is to apply enough temperature and pressure to ensure that the virgin UHMWPE particles are fully sintered. However, the virgin UHMWPE particles are not always sintered together well. The defects caused by incomplete consolidation or fusion of the UHMWPE powder are referred to as fusion defects. They have been associated with the presence of calcium stearate, which is used in some UHMWPE formulations to scavenge excess chemicals used in the polymerization process. Fusion defects greatly affect the mechanical properties of the UHMWPE and are thought to render the UHMWPE susceptible to fatigue failure and high rates of wear.

There are several different types of UHMWPE; some of the more common ones are GUR 4150 (pronounced as "G-U-R forty-one fifty"), GUR 4020, and GUR 4120, made by Hoechst Celanese, and Hylamer—made by DuPont. The Hoechst Celanese designations are coded by place of manufacture (4 = Texas, 1 = Europe), presence of calcium stearate (1 = present, 0 = free of calcium stearate), and pressure of formation (2 = low, 5 = high). The zero at the end has no meaning. Not all polyethylene is created equal; in fact, even the same lot of polyethylene can have very different properties, which can even be direction dependent within the same section.

16.4.2.2 Sterilization of UHMWPE

Gamma irradiation in air causes subsequent oxidation of UHMWPE. The oxidation process continues as the implant sits on the shelf before use and again after implantation. Oxidation is a form of chemical attack that leads to chain scission, effectively lowering molecular weight. A somewhat simplified approach to understanding oxidation and its effect on wear is to realize that the UHMWPE is becoming more like HDPE. HDPE has shorter chain lengths, is denser and more crystalline, and exhibits a higher wear rate than UHMWPE. High oxidation levels often mirror high levels of damage in vivo; however, more controlled studies are required to understand this problem fully. In the clinical scenario, not all implants that experience high wear rates exhibit debris-related failure. Similarly, some implants with very little apparent wear exhibit failure that would be associated with wear. With time, peak oxidation changes in UHMWPE due to gamma irradiation in air are found 1–2 mm below the surface of the implant. This subsurface region is commonly referred to as the "white band." Other types of UHMWPE sterilization under investigation are gamma irradiation in an inert environment (inert gas or vacuum [if there is no O_2 gas, there would be no oxidation]), ethylene oxide, and gas plasma.

Another effect of gamma irradiation in UHMWPE is cross-linking of polymer chains. Cross-linking of the chains should increase resistance to wear. Irradiation then creates both enhancement and reduction of the properties of UHMWPE simultaneously. Researchers are currently exploring methods of creating a high cross-link density in UHMWPE without also creating oxidation. Initial studies show tremendous increases in wear resistance with high-density cross-linking but decreases in fracture toughness and tensile strength. To understand the possible implications of such a new material, one must first be familiar with the types of UHMWPE wear found in orthopaedics.

16.4.2.3 Wear of UHMWPE in Total Joint Replacement

UHMWPE wear is a key factor that limits the performance of total hip and knee replacements. The problems with UHMWPE wear in the hip and knee are different and result in different clinical manifestations of wear. We present an overview of wear so that the reasons for these differences may be understood. This subject may wear on your patience, but bear with it; eventually it will become clear.

AN OVERVIEW OF WEAR.   There are three main aspects of the implant that may affect the generation of wear debris in total joint replacement: materials and manufacturing processes, implant design, and implant fixation. Only the aspect of materials and manufacturing processes are covered in this chapter.

Many primary factors affect wear, including material, load, contact type (sliding, rolling), motion type (unidirectional, reciprocating), motion velocity, motion cyclic frequency, track geometry (linear, path-crossing, etc.), lubricant rheology and chemistry, temperature, contact geometry, surface topography (roughness, texture), sliding distance, and number of cycles. These primary factors determine the dominant lubrication mechanism, lubricant flow and debris transport, local temperature and chemistry, and local stresses (their constraints and time dependence). These in turn determine the wear mechanism and failure mode (if any).

TYPES AND MODES OF WEAR MECHANISMS.   The three main types of wear mechanisms in total joint replacement are adhesive wear, abrasive wear, and fatigue wear. Adhesive wear occurs when the bonding between contact points exceeds the inherent strength of the UHMWPE. Adhesive wear results in formation of very small PE fibrils and a glossy surface; this wear type is often seen in acetabular components. Abrasive wear occurs when asperities on one surface are pressed into the opposite surface and plow scratches with articulation. In fatigue wear, cyclic stresses form small particles that are released as wear debris.

Four modes of wear occur in total joint replacement: 1) primary wear; 2) secondary, nonbearing surface wear; 3) third-body wear; and 4) nonbearing surface wear. The primary-wear mode occurs between two bearing surfaces that were intended to be in articulation, such as the UHMWPE tibial plateau and the cobalt-chromium-alloy femoral component. In secondary, nonbearing surface wear, a primary surface articulates against a surface never intended to be a bearing surface. Such would be the case if the UHMWPE of the patellar component wore through and the metal backing articulated with the femoral component. Third-body wear occurs when two primary bearing surfaces move with third-body particles trapped between them. A perfect example of third-body wear occurs when fragments of bone cement migrate into the synovial fluid and are trapped between the femoral component and the tibial plateau in the total knee replacement. Finally, nonbearing surface wear develops when motion occurs between two secondary, nonbearing surfaces. An example of nonbearing-surface wear might be the very slight movement of a UHMWPE tibial plateau against the metal tray.

CLINICAL RELEVANCE OF UHMWPE WEAR IN TOTAL HIP RE-PLACEMENT. In total hip arthroplasty, the mechanical aspects of wear account for only a minority of all clinical failures. The major clinical problem is the generation of many submicron-sized PE wear particles and their access to tissues. The very small particles incite a foreign-body inflammatory response and may lead to osteolysis. Studies indicate that patients with a high annual rate of UHMWPE wear in the acetabular cup and high rates of wear-debris generation have higher rates of osteolysis than those with lower rates of UHMWPE loss and debris generation. The submicron particles that are produced are often shaped like fibrils that seem to have been stretched; these particles are formed by the adhesive wear mechanism. The wear causes the surface of the UHMWPE to appear abraded or polished. The stresses generated in the UHMWPE in the total hip are mainly compressive. Because surface wear is the primary concern in total hip replacement, initial research results of the new high-density, cross-linked UHMWPE indicate that it may be a better material for use in the acetabular component. Much more research is required to prove this hypothesis.

CLINICAL RELEVANCE OF UHMWPE WEAR IN TOTAL KNEE REPLACEMENT.   Wear in the UHMWPE of the total knee replacement is better referred to as "wear damage." The types of PE damage mechanisms in the total knee components include adhesion, abrasion, burnishing, pitting, delamination, and fracture; the term *wear damage* encompasses all of these different phenomena. The numerous damage modes are probably due to the higher stresses and different kinematics (rolling/sliding) as compared to the hip. There is a widely accepted hypothesis that damage to polyethylene is a function of the stresses generated in use.

Have you ever considered why potholes form in city streets? Street potholes form for the same reason that the UHMWPE of tibial component in total knee replacement delaminates and pits. When car tires roll and slide (from braking) on city streets, both tensile and shear stresses are generated. The maximum shear stress is, however, located below the surface of the pavement. Similarly, in the UHMWPE of the tibial plateau, rolling and sliding cause maximum compression at the surface, tensile stresses tangential to the surface, and shear stresses that reach a maximum beneath the surface at a distance of approximately 1–2 mm. This is the same location as the "white band" that formed from gamma irradiation sterilization in air as shown in figure 16.12. The UHMWPE tibial component is in double jeopardy when gamma irradiated.

Due to this state of stress, the wear contribution in total knee components is mainly from fatigue. Cracks propagate through fatigue, causing pitting and delamination. Pits can be formed by propagation of cracks from the surface into the polyethylene to the region of the maximum shear stresses. They can also be produced by propagation of subsurface cracks (created by the maximum shear stress) up toward the surface. Extensive delamination occurs when the subsurface crack continues to propagate parallel to the surface, thus creating a partially detached layer of material. There are clinical manifestations of the different UHMWPE wear mechanisms in TKR as compared to THR. Osteolysis (which may be caused by the presence of the submicron-sized particles and not by the larger fatigue-wear particles) has a higher prevalence in THR than in TKR.

Unlike THR, UHMWPE wear of the tibial component in TKR is not primarily at the surface. The new high-density, cross-linked UHMWPE

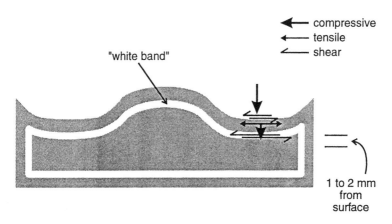

Figure 16.12. Because of the compression and the sliding and rolling mechanisms of loading in the knee, the polyethylene of the tibial component in total knee replacement is subjected to many different types of stress. In this schematic of a polyethylene tibial-bearing surface, one can see that the location of the maximum shear stress is below the contact surface in the material. The location of this stress coincides with the area of time-dependent material changes that can be induced through gamma irradiation.

may not be appropriate for use as a tibial plateau because of its reduced fracture toughness and tensile strength. Again, much more research is required to prove this statement.

Q16: Clinical Question (summary)

Pearl's plastic on the tibial side of her total knee component was badly worn. These modern plastic components should last forever, should they not? What happened to this one?

A16: Clinical Answer

As the old saying goes, "nothing lasts forever"! That statement is particularly true for ultrahigh molecular weight polyethylene. As discussed in Section 16.4.2.3, the rolling and sliding of the femoral component on the UHMWPE of the tibial component causes it to experience maximum compression at the surface, tensile stresses tangential to the surface, and shear stresses that reach a maximum beneath the surface at a distance of approximately 1–2 mm. It is very likely that the Pearl's tibial component had been sterilized with gamma irradiation. Progressively increasing oxidation probably followed, thus weakening the UHMWPE at the exact location of the maximum subsurface shear stress. The pitting and delamination found in the polyethylene is very likely related to this phenomenon.

Additional Reading

Aikins JL: *Wear Issues in Knees: Knee Design.* Technical Monograph 97-2000-145. Zimmer, Warsaw, Ind., 1995.

Black J: *Orthopaedic Biomaterials in Research and Practice.* Churchill Livingstone, New York, 1988.

Haas SS, Brauer GM, Dickson G: A characterization of polymethyl methacrylate bone cement. *J Bone Joint Surg* 57A(3):380–391, 1975.

Li S, Burstein AH: Ultra-high molecular weight polyethylene. The material and its use in total joint implants. *J Bone Joint Surg* 76A(7):1080–90, 1994.

Li S, Chang JD, Barrena EG, Furman BD, Wright TM, Salvati E: Nonconsolidated polyethylene particles and oxidation in Charnley acetabular cups. *Clin Orthop* 319:54–63, 1995.

Lin ST, Hawkins ME: *PMMA Precoating Technology.* Technical Monograph 97-2000-141. Zimmer, Warsaw, Ind., 1995.

Meyer PR, Lautenschlager EP, Moore BK: On the setting properties of acrylic bone cement. *J Bone Joint Surg* 55A(1):149–156, 1973.

Overview and Fundamentals of UHMWPE. Fact on UHMWPE: Part One of a Series on Ultra-High Molecular Weight Polyethylene. Technical Monograph 6092–0-009. Howmedica, Rutherford, N.J., 1994.

Park JB: *Biomaterials Science and Engineering.* Plenum, New York, 1984.

Ratner BD, Hoffman AS, Schoen FJ, Lemons JE (Eds): *Biomaterials Science: An Introduction to Materials in Medicine.* Academic Press, San Diego, 1996.

St. John KR (Ed): *Particulate Debris from Medical Implants: Mechanisms of Formation and Biological Consequences.* ASTM STP 1144, American Society for Testing and Materials, Philadelphia, 1992.

17

Tissue Mechanics

CLINICAL SCENARIO: TEAR OF THE PATELLAR TENDON

Arrowhead Stadium was the site of the umpteenth meeting of the Kansas City Chiefs and their arch rivals, the Oakland Raiders. Kansas City returned the kickoff to their own 28-yard line and, determined to strike early and often, sent their prime wide receiver on a long down and out into Raider territory. Just as the receiver caught the ball, he was hit by two Oakland defenders, and his knee flexed acutely. The receiver felt an immediate burning pain in the front of his knee and was unable to stand up again. Examination in the locker room by the team physician revealed a high-riding patella and a palpable depression where the patellar tendon normally resided. How could such a well-conditioned athlete sustain a tendon rupture?

The materials found naturally in our body are by far the most fascinating structural materials on this earth. Our tissues are constantly changing, adapting to their environment, and repairing themselves. Would it not be nice to have an airplane made out of a self-repairing material when a crack starts to form in a wing? Perhaps someday there will be such artificially intelligent synthetic materials, but for now, only our own bodies can perform such miraculous feats. The extraordinary qualities of tissues, however, make them difficult to study and characterize as materials. In this chapter, we present information about bone, tendon, ligament, and cartilage, and we attempt to explain the general mechanical function and design of these tissues.

■ 17.1 VISCOELASTIC NATURE OF TISSUES

Up to this point, the materials discussed in this primer have all been solids or at least treated as solids. In tissues, however, the fluidlike behavior of the material must be considered. Most soft tissues (and some polymers) that act partly like solids and partly like fluids are said to be viscoelastic or to exhibit viscoelastic behavior. Ligament, tendon, cartilage, fascia, and, to a limited degree, bone are all examples of viscoelastic materials.

17.1.1 Mechanical Models of Viscoelastic Behavior

Small, imaginary mechanical devices that model viscoelastic behavior can be quite helpful. In chapter 3 we learned that a spring is a very faithful analog of elastic behavior. Similarly, viscous behavior can be modeled by a piston in a piston chamber, which collectively is often called a dash pot. A plunger in a hypodermic syringe is a good example of a dash pot. Both a spring and a dash pot are shown in figure 17.1. If a force is applied to pull out the plunger, the surrounding fluid (e.g., air) leaks into the syringe around the plunger, and the plunger moves a distance Δl over a time period Δt. The rate of movement, $\Delta l / \Delta t$, is proportional to the applied force and can be written as $F = \mu \, (\Delta l / \Delta t)$, where μ is a constant analogous to the viscosity (or thickness) of a fluid.

A simple viscoelastic material can be modeled by putting a spring and a dash pot in series (figure 17.2a). Such an arrangement is called a Maxwell body. If a force F is applied to this system (figure 17.2b) and maintained for a period of time, the displacement over the course of time is shown in figure 17.2c. At the time t_o when the force is first applied, the spring elongates instantaneously by an amount d_s. Because plunger movement is time dependent, it makes no contribution to this initial, *instantaneous* displacement. Thereafter, as time passes, the dash pot adds to the displacement continuously, and the overall displacement continues to increase. If the load is removed at time t_1, the spring will contract, and the displacement will be reduced by the amount d_s, but, because no force is acting, there is no reason for the plunger to return to its original position, so the displacement produced by viscous flow will persist beyond time t_1.

An alternative arrangement puts the spring and dash pot in parallel

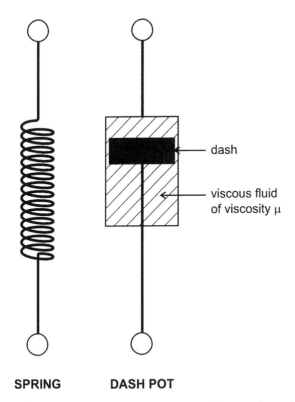

SPRING   **DASH POT**

Figure 17.1. The spring and the dash pot are the two elements used to make models of viscoelastic behavior.

(figure 17.3a). This model is called a Kelvin body. When an instantaneous load is applied to this system, there is no instantaneous movement because the spring cannot elongate unless there is an equal displacement of the dash pot plunger, and a dash pot cannot exhibit instantaneous movement (figure 17.3b). Thereafter, the displacement occurs continuously over time with the spring supporting an increasing proportion of the load as it extends. Eventually the spring approaches its maximum extension (for the applied load) and at this point is carrying almost all the load. Because there is now little force acting on the dash pot, its movement is very slow, and the displacement of the system approaches a constant value. If the load is removed at a later time, t_1, the spring will begin to contract against the dash pot, and the dis-

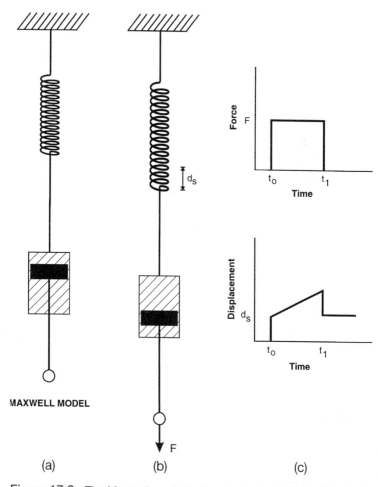

Figure 17.2. The Maxwell model is the simplest representation of viscoelastic behavior. The spring responds instantly to the applied force, whereas the dash pot deforms gradually with time.

placement will be completely reversed; the system thus returns to its original configuration. Neither Maxwell nor Kelvin bodies have been found to be good models for the mechanical behavior of various types of connective tissue.

A somewhat more complex system is shown in figure 17.4a, in which a spring is placed in series with a subunit that is itself a Kelvin

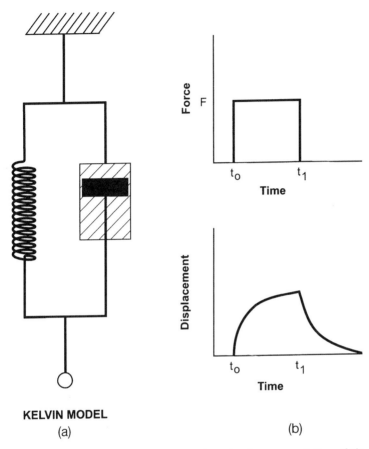

KELVIN MODEL

(a)   (b)

Figure 17.3. The Kelvin model is another simple representation of viscoelastic behavior. When the spring and dash pot are put in parallel,
they must experience equal displacements, so the dash pot controls
the rate of response to an applied load.

body. In this case, application of the load at time t_o produces instantaneous displacement because of the stretching of spring S_2 (region I, figure 17.4b). Thereafter, displacement of the dash pot and spring S_1 behaves as in figure 17.3, so that there is a continuous increase in
displacement after t_o (region II) in addition to the instantaneous displacement. If the force is removed at time t_1, spring S_2 will contract instantaneously (region III), and thereafter spring S_1 will cause contrac-

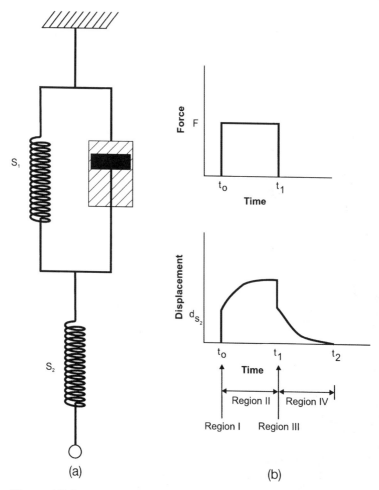

Figure 17.4. A more complex model of viscoelastic behavior puts a spring in series with a spring and dash pot in parallel. This is more realistic than the simple Kelvin and Maxwell models.

tion of the Kelvin body (region IV) until time t_2, when all of the displacement has been recovered. Although many more complicated arrangements are possible, this three-component model is a relatively good analog for the behavior of many structural tissues such as ligaments, tendons, and bone.

17.1.2 Characteristics of Viscoelastic Material Behavior

Viscoelastic behavior implies a time-dependent behavior in a material. Viscoelastic materials exhibit three basic characteristics not displayed in other materials. These are strain-rate-dependent properties, creep, and stress relaxation. Each of these phenomena is discussed separately in the following sections.

17.1.2.1 Strain-Rate-Dependent Properties

In an actual tensile test, the load is not raised from zero to a finite level instantaneously; rather, it is applied over a short, but definite, period of time. For this reason, a small amount of viscous flow occurs during the initial apparent elastic displacement. The rate at which the specimen is displaced is referred to as the stroke rate, and the corresponding rate of change of strain is the strain rate. In general, biological materials appear to be stiffer when stretched at high strain rates and softer if pulled at lower strain rates. Because of this, whenever stiffness data (modulus of elasticity) are reported for polymeric or tissue materials, the strain rate used in the test should always be given.

> In general, the faster a tissue is stretched, the stiffer it will appear to be.

Interestingly, as the strain rate increases, viscoelastic materials in general become stronger; that is, the stress at fracture increases. The elongation to fracture decreases, however. An example of this type of behavior is given for cortical bone in the longitudinal direction. At low strain rates, bone specimens elongate considerably (several percent) before fracture, whereas at high strain rates, bone acts more like a purely brittle material for which the deformation to fracture is mostly elastic. Other materials also behave in this fashion. An extreme example is the child's and physical therapist's entertainment medium called Silly Putty. At strain rates of about an inch per minute, a "cigar" of Silly Putty can be extended to a length of several feet while thinning down to a threadlike diameter before breaking. This same "cigar" of Silly Putty will break in a truly brittle fashion if the ends are jerked apart as rapidly as one's hands can move. In this model experiment, it is also easy to detect that the resistance to fracture (i.e., the strength of the Silly Putty) is very much greater at the high strain rates than at the low. Have a little fun and prove this concept to yourself firsthand!

> ➢ In general, viscoelastic materials such as tissues exhibit higher loads to fracture with less elongation when stretched faster.

17.1.2.2 Creep

When a viscoelastic specimen is subjected to a constant and continuously maintained load (as illustrated in figure 17.5), there is an initial elongation due to the elastic response, and this is followed by a viscous component of flow known as *creep,* or cold flow.

Cold flow is experienced by high-density polyethylene acetabular prosthesis when subjected to joint loads in total hip arthroplasty. This cold flow contributes to the decrease in the superior wall thickness of the cup, which can be deduced from radiographs over time. Note that this decrease is also due in part to the actual loss of material caused by wear of the prosthesis, so it is difficult to determine from the radiographs alone how much thinning is due to wear and how much is due to cold flow.

> ➢ *Creep* is the continuous deformation of a viscoelastic material over time when a constant load is applied.

17.1.2.3 Stress Relaxation

In a similar experiment, a viscoelastic specimen can be extended rapidly by an amount Δl and held at the new length. The strain, which is constant throughout the test, is $\varepsilon = \Delta l / l_o$. A load cell in series with the specimen will detect the force necessary to produce this displacement (figure 17.6). After the initial elongation at t_o, the force required to maintain the constant strain decreases continuously with time. This is known as *stress relaxation.*

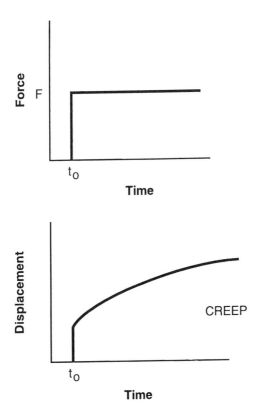

Figure 17.5. Creep behavior in a viscoelastic material is gradual deformation with time under an applied load.

A clinically relevant example of stress relaxation is the tensioning of a Teflon or Dacron prosthetic anterior cruciate ligament (ACL) during knee reconstruction. At surgery, the prosthesis is loaded to a certain predetermined level and is then fixed between the components of the knee. The force with which the prosthetic ligament draws the femur and the tibia together then decreases over a period of hours due to stress relaxation within the polymeric prosthesis. Because of this, the contraction forces initially imposed on the joint cannot be maintained for any significant period of time.

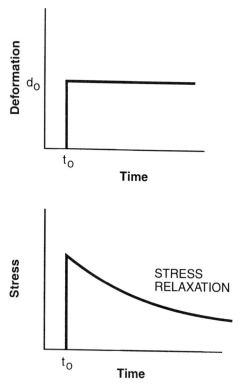

Figure 17.6. Stress relaxation in a viscoelastic material is the gradual reduction in stress with time with a constant applied deformation.

> ➤ Stress relaxation is the decrease in stress with time in a viscoelastic specimen under constant strain.

Both creep and stress relaxation behavior can be assessed quantitatively using conventional mechanical testing techniques. Together, these two tests can be used to characterize the viscoelastic behavior of various tissues and polymers under a variety of loading and strain-rate conditions.

17.2 BONE

Bone is found in many different forms in the body. The most fundamental distinction for bone is whether it is cortical or cancellous. These
two general categories of bone have very different mechanical properties and are covered separately in this text.

17.2.1 Cortical Bone

There are several different types of cortical bone. The type formed in
the body depends on the age, location, growth rate, and stress conditions during development. Our discussion focuses only on the properties of osteonal compact bone.

Compact or cortical bone is a complex structure of organized osteons
held together with less organized matrix. The mineral or inorganic
phase comprises about 60–70 weight percent of bone. Water makes up
about 5%–8% of bone, and the remainder is extracellular organic matrix material. The extracellular organic matrix material is about 90%
type I collagen.

The compact bone found in long bones is generally considered to be
transversely isotropic, meaning that it has about the same properties in
all directions of the transverse plane (that is, it is isotropic in the transverse plane) and significantly different properties in the longitudinal direction. In fact, the stiffness and strength in the longitudinal direction
can be about one and a half times greater than in the transverse direction. This directional dependence of properties can be easily understood by considering the directional organization of the cortical bone.
The osteons are lined up in the longitudinal direction and strengthen
and stiffen the bone along their length. Conversely, in the transverse
plane, the less-organized matrix controls the properties of the bone.
Typical values of strength and stiffness of cortical bone in the transverse and longitudinal directions are given in table 17.1.

> ➣ Cortical bone is often considered to be
> transversely isotropic in mechanical prop-
> erties.

Table 17.1   Typical properties of cortical bone in the longitudinal and transverse directions

Property	Longitudinal	Transverse
Elastic modulus	14–24 GPa	8–18 GPa
Tensile strength	130 MPa	50 MPa
Compressive strength	190 MPa	130 MPa

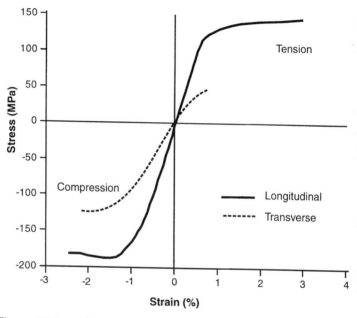

Figure 17.7. Cortical bone is stronger and stiffer in the longitudinal direction as compared to the transverse orientation. It also exhibits different mechanical properties in tension and compression. *Adapted from:* Gibson LJ and Ashby MF: *Cellular Solids: Structure & Properties.* Pergamon Press, Oxford, England, 1988, p. 320, figure 11.4.

Figure 17.7 shows typical stress-strain data for cortical bone in the longitudinal and transverse directions in both tension and compression. Notice that not only are the stiffnesses and loads to failure lower in the transverse orientation, but the energy to failure and ductility are also substantially less. How does this information tie together with the failure mechanisms of bone presented in chapter 9?

Bone is a living tissue that remodels continuously throughout a person's life and adapts to the mechanical conditions to which it is subjected. This process is defined by Wolff's law (see chapter 6). Remodeling in bone is a surface phenomenon that occurs on periosteal, endosteal, haversian canal, and trabecular surfaces. Even in the elderly, cortical remodeling rates can be as high as 2%–5% per year.

Stress fractures in bone are the fatigue damage that accumulates due to high stresses applied over shorter periods of time. Under conditions of normal activity, any fatigue damage caused by imposed stresses is repaired by remodeling of the (fatigue) microcracks. When repetitive high stresses are present, the rate of remodeling cannot keep up with the rate of microcrack formation, and stress fractures result. Stress fractures are relatively common in long-distance runners, race horses, and military personnel who undergo rigorous training.

The stiffness and strength of cortical bone progressively decrease with age after early adulthood. Studies estimate that the fracture energy of cortical bone decreases about 7% per decade. In general, with aging, normal nondiseased human bone becomes less stiff, less strong, and more brittle.

Osteoporosis is a disease state that causes a decrease in bone mass with a decrease in density. This results in fragility or decrease in strength of the bone. Osteoporosis can be induced through metabolic changes (particularly in older women), certain nutritional deficiencies, excessive use of alcohol, and disuse. Osteomalacia is the disease state characterized by the softening of bone. In this disease, the bone mass is not necessarily decreased, but the degree of mineralization is lowered.

Cortical bone displays viscoelastic characteristics of creep, stress relaxation, and strain-rate dependency. As an example, figure 17.8 shows typical stress-strain data for cortical bone in the longitudinal direction at different strain rates. As this graph shows, the apparent stiffness, strength, and toughness of bone is a function of the imposed strain rate. Typical strain rates experienced by the body are 0.001/second under slow walking, 0.01/second under brisk walking, 0.03/second with slow running and much higher strain rates under impact loading. The maximum energy-absorption capacity is from 0.01 to 0.1/second strain rates, which coincides with the normal range of strenuous activities.

17.2.2 Cancellous Bone

The schematics in figure 17.9 illustrate the three different, basic architectures of cancellous bone: rod-rod, plate-plate, and plate-rod. The dif-

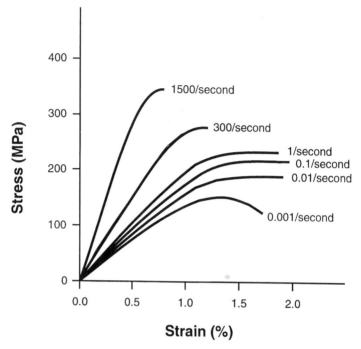

Figure 17.8. Bone is a viscoelastic material that exhibits strain-rate-dependent apparent stiffnesses and fracture energies. In this test of cortical bone in the longitudinal direction, the energy to failure is maximum at normal physiological strain rates. *Adapted from:* McElhaney JH: Dynamic response of bone and muscle tissue. *J Applied Physiology* 21:1231, 1966, p. 1233, figure 5.

ferent structures form in response to the environment and mechanical loads imposed during development. For example, the rod-rod architecture forms in areas in which nearly equal stresses are imposed in all directions, whereas the plate-plate structure forms in response to very directional stresses. Cancellous bone can be either nearly isotropic or very anisotropic, depending on the architecture.

Because of its porous nature, cancellous bone is much weaker and much less stiff than cortical bone. The stiffness of cancellous bone can range from 0.010 to 2.0 GPa. The stiffness and strength of cancellous bone depends on its orientation and density. For the rod-rod architecture, for example, the strength and stiffness can be related to the square

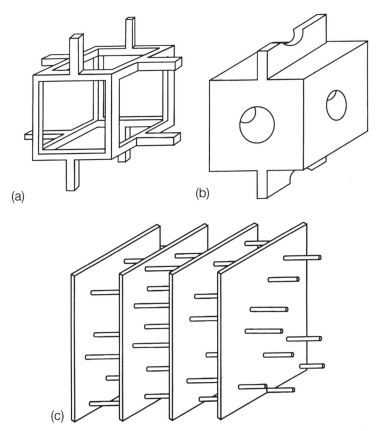

Figure 17.9. Several models represent the different forms of cancellous bone. *(a)* The rod-rod structure represents the less dense, more isotropic cancellous bone. *(b)* The plate-plate structure is denser and yet random, and *(c)* the rod-plate structure is dense and more anisotropic. *Adapted from:* Gibson LJ and Ashby MF: *Cellular Solids: Structure & Properties.* Pergamon Press, Oxford, England, 1988, p. 327, figure 11.12.

of the relative density. Different relationships are estimated for other architectures.

The viscoelastic response of cancellous bone is very dependent on the marrow or fluid that fills its open spaces. Cancellous bone is stiffer and tougher when marrow is present. The hydrodynamic effects of marrow are very important in protecting bone (particularly in impact loading).

■ 17.3 ARTICULAR CARTILAGE

Articular cartilage protects bone from high stresses and provides a low-friction bearing surface for the joint. In fact, the combination of healthy, normal, articular cartilage surfaces with synovial fluid lubrication equals the best synthetic bearings. In this section, we study the form and function of both normal and damaged articular cartilage.

> ➤ The healthy joint articulation has extremely good bearing surface characteristics as compared to human-made designs.

Articular cartilage is composed of an extracellular matrix throughout which chondrocytes are dispersed. The extracellular matrix consists of proteoglycans, collagens, water, and other proteins and glycoproteins. The concentration and distribution of these components vary throughout the depth of the cartilage and are related to the function of the cartilage.

There are four major depth zones of articular cartilage (figure 17.10). In the *superficial zone* (at the articulating surface), the collagen fibrils are arranged parallel to the surface, there is a relatively low proteoglycan content, the condrocytes are elongated along the surface, and the highest water content (about 80%) occurs. The alignment of the collagen fibrils provides this layer with the tensile strength required to resist the stretching created during surface contact. During initial loading, the high water content of the superficial zone permits initial compressive creep due to fluid exudation.

The *transition* (or *middle*) zone is composed of large-diameter collagen fibrils and more rounded chondrocytes that are less organized than in the superficial zone. The *deep zone* has the highest proteoglycan content and the lowest water content (about 65%). In the deep zone, the collagen fibers are of large diameter and are oriented perpendicular to the surface; the chondrocytes are nearly spherical and are arranged in columns. Although not as stiff in tension, the middle and deep zones govern the shear behavior of cartilage. The randomly dispersed collagen fibrils stretch and entrap the proteoglycans during shear.

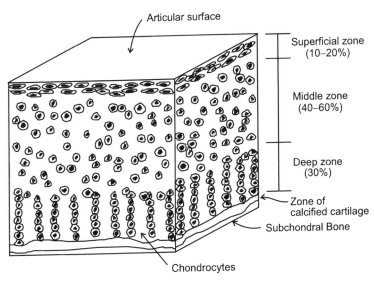

Figure 17.10. This schematic of the cross-section of articular cartilage shows the variation in structure throughout the depth. *Adapted from: Basic Biomechanics of the Musculoskeletal System*, 2nd ed., M Nordin and VH Frankel, Eds. Lea & Febiger, Philadelphia, 1989, p. 32, figure 2-1.

The fourth zone is the *zone of calcified cartilage,* which separates hyaline cartilage from subchondral bone. In this layer, the chondrocytes are more rounded, and there is less organization, which provides a good transition to the underlying bone.

As stated previously, a main function of articular cartilage is to protect the bone from high stresses. Cartilage does this by reducing the maximum contact stress and distributing the stresses more evenly to the bone. The stiffness of cartilage is about 1/20 that of subchondral cancellous bone and 1/65 that of cortical bone. The cartilage therefore deforms much more than bone under the same applied loads. Similar to a water bed, it fills in incongruities and spreads the load over the articulating surface in order to increase contact area and therefore decrease contact stress.

➤ Articular cartilage protects bone from high stresses.

We can best understand the properties and load-distributing characteristics of cartilage by considering it as a biphasic material, that is, as a material with a solid phase and a fluid phase. The collagen fibrils form a strong, fatigue-resistant matrix in which proteoglycans (and other constituents) exert pressure. Water is an important constituent in cartilage for many reasons. The hydrophilic proteoglycans swell in the presence of water and provide rigidity in the collagen network matrix. In fact, the viscoelastic behavior of cartilage is governed by the rate at which fluid may be forced out of the tissue. When subjected to a compressive force (such as a joint reaction force), healthy cartilage will deform gradually with time as fluid slowly flows out (figure 17.11). Similarly, stress relaxation in cartilage occurs through the gradual redistribution of the fluids and other constituents.

In disease states, changes occur in the cartilage composition that alter its mechanical properties. For example, in osteoarthritis, changes in the cartilage are initially mechanically induced either by trauma or more gradually over a period of time. This initial damage results in a decrease in proteoglycans, which increases the water concentration in the structures and increases permeability to water. The loss of the rigidity provided by the proteoglycans makes the cartilage less able to withstand and distribute loads to the underlying bone. The amount of decrease in proteoglycans can be directly related to the severity of the osteoarthritis.

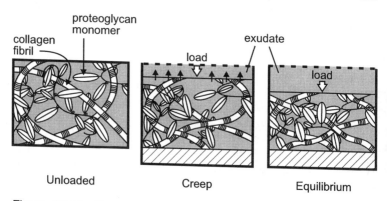

Figure 17.11. This schematic shows the creep response of cartilage when a constant stress is applied. Creep continues until equilibrium is reached. *Adapted from:* Armstrong CG and Mow VC: Friction, Lubrication and Wear of Synovial Joints. In *Scientific Foundations of Orthopaedics and Traumatology,* R Owen, J Goodfellow, and P Bullough, Eds. William Heinemann Medical Books Inc., London, 1980, pp. 223–232, figure 1.

■ 17.4 KNEE MENISCUS

The meniscus distributes forces in the knee throughout its range of motion. Studies estimate that the meniscus carries 50% of the joint reaction force in extension and 85%–90% in flexion. Without the meniscus, there is a 50%–70% increase in peak contact stresses. The meniscus also acts as a shock absorber, attenuating the dynamic stresses generated at heel strike by as much as 20%.

The meniscus is composed of about 26 weight percent solids (collagen, proteoglycans, and other proteins) and 74 weight percent fluids (water and electrolytes). The solid phase is porous and permeable, so the fluids of the meniscus can aid in lubrication of the knee joint.

The structure and organization of the solid phase of the meniscus provides it with the strength required to bear a high proportion of the joint reaction forces. Figure 17.12 shows a simple schematic of the meniscus organization. The collagen fibrils are aligned both diagonally and circumferentially; the alignment of the collagen allows the meniscus to withstand the hoop tensile stresses created by the compressive joint reaction force.

■ 17.5 TENDONS

Primarily because of their collagen fiber composition and arrangement, tendons have the highest tensile strength of any soft tissue. The major constituent of a tendon is collagen, which is about 86% of its dry weight. Tendons exhibit various levels of organization in which collagen fibrils are embedded in a matrix of proteoglycans and cells. The mechanical properties and behavior of tendons depend on the properties and architecture of the components. Figure 17.13 illustrates the general architecture of a tendon, and figure 17.14 shows typical load-displacement behavior of a tendon in tension. Small bundles of aligned collagen fibers form larger bundles of fibrils that eventually form the tendon. Crimping of the collagen fibrils allows the tendon to have an initial low stiffness, usually referred to as the toe region. As the crimping straightens out, the stiffness of the tendon increases rapidly; the slope of this linear region is usually used to represent the elastic modulus of the tendon. Finally, failure of tendons occurs when the collagen fibrils tear and separate.

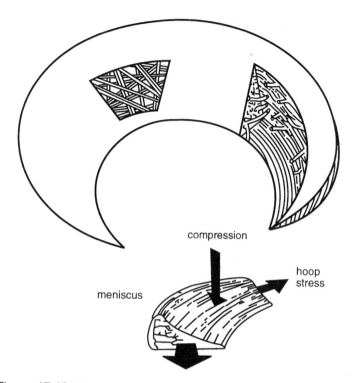

Figure 17.12. The meniscus is a complex mechanical structure designed to resist compression and hoop stresses. *Adapted from:* Fithian DC, Kelly MA, Mow VC: Material properties and structure-function relationships in the menisci. *Clinical Orthopaedics and Related Research* 252:19–31, 1990, p. 22, figure 2.

Tendons are viscoelastic in nature; they exhibit stress relaxation, creep, and hysteresis. Hysteresis is the loss of energy upon recovery of strain. Tendons recover much (90%–96% per cycle) of the elastic strain energy and therefore waste little energy during activity. During repeated loading and unloading, tendons do gradually increase in strain at a given stress level. About 10 loading and unloading cycles are required to achieve repeatable results. Tendons are also sensitive to the rate of testing. Higher strain rates make the tendon stiffer; however, this effect is not as pronounced as with other soft tissues. The age of the tendon affects its mechanical properties as well. Stiffness and ultimate stress of the tendon increase up to skeletal maturity.

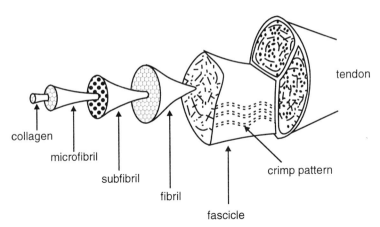

collagen

microfibril

subfibril

fibril

fascicle

crimp pattern

tendon

Figure 17.13. The tendon has many different levels of organization. *Adapted from:* Kastelic J, Galeski A, Baer E: The multi-composite structure of tendon. *Connect. Tissue Res.* 6:11–23, 1978, p. 21, figure 27.

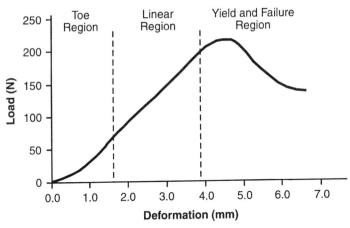

Figure 17.14. Typical load-displacement behavior of a tendon in tension.

■ 17.6 LIGAMENTS

Ligaments are dense connective tissues that are grossly and microscopically similar to tendons. Ligaments differ from tendons by having a lower percentage of collagen, a higher percentage of ground substance, and a more random organization of collagen. The tensile-load-elongation behavior of ligaments is nonlinear as shown in a typical curve in

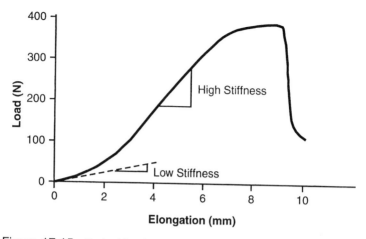

Figure 17.15. Typical load-elongation curve of a ligament in tension.

figure 17.15. There is a low-stiffness region and a high-stiffness region in this curve. The low-stiffness region is a result of the straightening out of the undulating pattern of collagen. When the undulations are straightened out, the stretching fibrils then resist the load more forcefully and produce the higher stiffness behavior.

Ligaments are also viscoelastic in nature because of the interaction of the collagen and ground substance. Ligaments exhibit creep, stress relaxation, strain rate sensitivity, and hysteresis. The load-elongation response of ligaments depends on the history of loading (figure 17.16); the apparent stiffness depends on previous loadings. Similarly, ligaments have higher apparent ultimate loads and absorbed energy at high strain rates as compared to low rates.

This behavior has several clinical implications. For example, in autogenous ACL reconstruction, the initial force applied to tension the graft decreases over time due to stress relaxation. The forces in the graft can decline by as much as 80% of the initial values in younger patients. Similarly, in spinal distraction, the displacement should be applied in small steps separated by a few minutes. Studies show that the peak forces applied to the instrumentation and its insertions on the vertebrae can be reduced by over 50% if time is allowed for creep of the vertebral ligaments and other soft tissues.

Several other factors affect the mechanical properties of ligaments. Ligaments have manyfold increases in stiffness, ultimate force, and en-

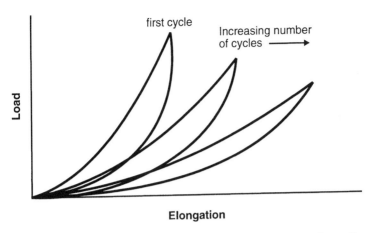

Figure 17.16. Typical loading and unloading curves in cyclic testing of knee ligaments. The load-elongation response of ligaments depends on the history of loading.

ergy absorbed with skeletal maturation. However, the stiffness and ultimate load for young-adult anterior cruciate ligaments can be more than three times greater than for ligaments from older individuals.

Immobilization is generally detrimental to ligament mechanical properties. Studies demonstrate that immobilization causes a decrease in ultimate tensile load, energy absorption, and elastic modulus. Typical load-displacement behavior before and after immobilization is shown in figure 17.17. These decreases are caused by a combination of changes to the insertions and in the ligament substance. Remobilization enables a slow reversal of mechanical properties. Studies indicate that rates of reversal range from 100% at nine weeks to 80%–90% at one year, depending on the location of the ligament.

Q17: Clinical Question (Summary)

The rivalry between the Kansas City Chiefs and the Oakland Raiders is always vicious, and this year is no exception. The Kansas City Chief's star wide receiver was hit by two Oakland defenders and suffered a severe patellar tendon rupture. How could such a well-conditioned athlete sustain a tendon rupture?

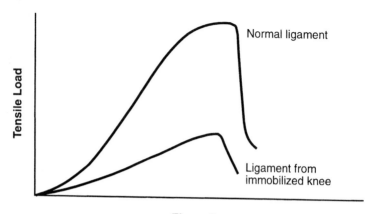

Figure 17.17. Typical load-displacement data for ligaments before and after immobilization. Immobilization of a ligament results in a decrease in load to failure and energy to failure.

A17: CLINICAL ANSWER

As in any material, there is a point beyond which integrity is lost. The impact on the football player was applied rapidly (Section 17.5), resulting in fiber rupture and, finally, total rupture of the tendon (figure 17.14).

Additional Reading

Carter DR: Mechanical loading history and skeletal biology. *J Biomech* 20(11/12):1095–1109, 1987.

Cochran GVB: *A Primer of Orthopaedic Biomechanics.* Churchill Livingstone, New York, 1982.

Fung YC: *Mechanical Properties of Living Tissues.* New York, Springer-Verlag, 1981.

Gibson LJ, Ashby MF: *Cellular Solids: Structure and Properties.* Pergamon Press, Oxford, England, 1988. Mow VC, Hayes WC (Eds): *Basic Orthopaedic Biomechanics.* Raven, New York, 1991.

Nordin M, Frankel VH (Eds): *Basic Biomechanics of the Musculoskeletal System,* 2d ed. Lea & Febiger, Philadelphia, 1989.

Glossary

Alloy   A metallic substance composed of two or more elements in solution

Annealing   High-temperature treatment (of alloys) that removes the effects of cold working and causes precipitates to go into solution

Anode   The electrode that undergoes corrosion in a galvanic cell; the negative electrode

Area moment of inertia, I   A geometrical property of the cross-sectional area of a structure that describes how the spatial distribution of material in the structure resists bending. Sometimes called the second moment. A mathematical unit, I is always determined in relation to some reference line, usually the neutral axis. Units: meters^4 or inches^4

Bending rigidity (EI)   Ability of a structure to resist bending; depends on spatial distribution of material in structure (I) and on the tensile stiffness (E) of the material of which the structure is made

Bending stress   Stress generated in structure due to an applied moment; does not depend on material

Brittle   A type of material failure that is preceded by little or no plastic deformation

Cantilever   A projecting beam or structural member supported at only one end

Cathode   The positive electrode in a galvanic cell

Cold flow   Creep in polymers at normal temperatures (e.g., cold flow in UHMWPE acetabular components)

Corrosion   Deterioration of a material because of interaction with its environment

Couple   A pure moment created by two forces of equal magnitude and opposite direction acting at equal distances from an axis of rotation

Creep   Continuing deformation of material (with time) under constant applied load (viscoelastic behavior)

Crevice corrosion   Corrosion in crevices where the oxygen tension becomes low, thus inhibiting the repair of the passive layer

Crystal   A material whose constituent atoms are arranged in an orderly pattern that repeats indefinitely in three dimensions

Deformation   Change in shape due to an applied force

Ductile   Capable of undergoing considerable plastic deformation

Ductility   Total plastic strain to failure of material. Units: percent

Elastic deformation   Recoverable or nonpermanent change in shape

Elasticity   Springiness; property of a body by which it regains its original shape after being deformed; behavior of perfectly elastic material

Endurance limit   Stress at which material can be cyclically loaded (fatigued) indefinitely without breaking

Energy   Ability to perform work. Units: newtons-meters or inches-pounds, 1 N m = 1 J (joule)

Fatigue   Of materials, the process of repeatedly applying loads that are too small to produce fracture in one application

Fatigue failure   Failure of material due to repetitive loading at stresses below the fracture strength

Force   "Push" or "pull" that accelerates a mass or deforms a structure. Units: newtons or pounds

Forged   Shaped by hammering

Fracture strength   Stress at which material breaks

Fretting   Rubbing

Fretting corrosion   Accelerated corrosion due to continual rubbing in multicomponent devices

Galvanic corrosion   Electrochemical corrosion process that occurs when two dissimilar metals are placed in contact in the presence of a corroding (electrolyte) medium

Grains   Microscopic crystals that make up metals, alloys, and ceramics

Kinetic energy   Energy of motion

Mass moment of inertia   Relates to dynamic motion of a body; describes resistance to angular acceleration

Mer   The chemical unit or molecule of which polymers are composed

Metal corrosion   Slow oxidation of metal in contact with water, usually an aerated saline solution

Modulus of elasticity or **elastic modulus** or **Young's modulus** *(E)*   Stiffness of a material under normal stress (tension or compression); slope of stress-strain curve; the quantity E in Hooke's law, $\sigma = E\varepsilon$. Units: newtons per square meter or pounds per square inch

Moment   Force applied at a distance from an axis of rotation. Units: newton-meters or pound-inches

Moment arm   Perpendicular distance from line of action of force to the pivot point or axis of rotation

Normal force   Force applied perpendicular to surface

Passivation   Formation of a thin adherent layer of corrosion products (oxides) on the surface of a metal that separates the metal from the solution and slows or prevents corrosion

Plastic deformation   Permanent or nonrecoverable change in shape

Plasticity   Property of a body by which it undergoes permanent deformation; behavior of material in plastic (or permanent) deformation

Polar moment of inertia, J   A geometrical property of the cross-sectional area of a structure that describes how the spatial distribution of material in the structure acts to resist twisting. J is always determined in relation to the torsion axis. Units: meters^4 or inches^4

Poisson's ratio   The ratio of a tensile specimen's contractile (radial) strain to its axial strain (elongation)

Polymer   A large molecule composed of a number of small chemical units, or mers

Potential energy   Stored energy available for use

Shear force   Force applied parallel to surface

Shear modulus (G)   Stiffness of material under shear loading. Units: newtons per square meter or pounds per square inch

Static equilibrium Situation where forces and moments are balanced, no motion occurs: $\Sigma F = 0$, $\Sigma M_o = 0$

Stiffness Relationship between stress and strain in an elastic material

Strain Change in shape normalized to original shape; dimensionless

Strain energy Energy stored in an elastically deformed material

Strain rate sensitivity The characteristic of a material whereby its stiffness (modulus) increases with increasing strain rate

Strength Stress at which a material fails

Stress Internal normalized forces that resist deformation. Units: force per area (pascals = newtons per square meter, or pounds per square inch)

Stress concentrations (stress raisers) Discontinuities in structures that lead to locally high stresses

Stress relaxation Reduction of stress in material (with time) under fixed deformation (viscoelastic behavior)

Stress corrosion Accelerated corrosion at highly stressed (therefore high-energy) regions

Torque Twisting moment. Units: newtons-meters or pounds-inches

Torsional rigidity (GJ) Ability of a structure to resist torsion; depends on spatial distribution of material in structure (J) and on the shear stiffness, G, of the material of which the structure is made

Toughness Work to fracture a material; area under load-deformation or stress-strain curve

Ultimate tensile strength Maximum stress in material during a single loading cycle to failure

Viscoelasticity The property of certain materials by which they exhibit a combination of instantaneous recoverable (elastic) and time-dependent, permanent (viscous) deformation

Work Force acting over a distance. Units: newton-meters or foot-pounds or inch-pounds

Wrought Shaped by plastic deformation; said of metals and alloys

Yield strength Stress at which a material yields or exhibits first permanent deformation

Questions Similar to Those of the OITE and Board

1. Cortical bone is anisotropic because

    a. It is a nonhomogeneous material.

    b. It is a viscoelastic material.

    c. Its material properties are different in different directions.

    d. It is subjected to many different types of loads and moments.

    e. It is a living tissue.

2. Strain in a metal that is not recovered upon release of the applied load is called

    a. Elastic deformation.

    b. Stress relaxation.

    c. Plastic deformation.

    d. Yield strength.

    e. Endurance limit.

3. With the elbow in full extension, a weight in the hand can be elevated by abduction of the whole arm. To do this, the muscle force across the shoulder must increase continually. This increasing muscle force will

    a. Decrease the joint reaction force but will overcome an increasing moment.

    b. Overcome an increasing moment only.

    c. Overcome a decreasing moment only.

    d. Increase the joint reaction force and overcome an increasing moment.

    e. Increase the joint reaction force only.

4. In mechanical characterization of a material, the change in deformation with time in response to a constant applied force is referred to as
   a. Ductility
   b. Elastic modulus
   c. Creep
   d. Ultimate tensile strength
   e. Toughness

5. One of the typical characteristics of a viscoelastic material is that
   a. It always exhibits linear elastic behavior.
   b. Its apparent material properties change with the rate of loading.
   c. Its yield strength is always greater than its ultimate tensile strength.
   d. Its mechanical properties are not temperature dependent.
   e. It degrades rapidly when implanted in the body.

6. If a prosthesis with a long neck is used in total hip arthroplasty, the distance from the abductor insertion to the center of rotation of the hip will be increased. The biomechanical consequences of this are to
   a. Decrease both the abduction moment arm and the body-weight moment arm.
   b. Decrease the abductor moment arm but leave the body-weight moment arm unchanged.
   c. Increase the abductor moment arm but leave the body-weight moment arm unchanged.
   d. Increase both the abductor moment arm and the body-weight moment arm.
   e. Increase the abductor moment arm but decrease the body-weight moment arm.

■ ANSWERS

1. Cortical bone is anisotropic because
   c. Its material properties are different in different directions.
      Materials that display different material properties in different directions are called anisotropic (see Section 3.5.1). As discussed in detail in Section 17.2.1, the compact bone found in long bones has significantly different properties along the long axis as compared with those of the transverse plane. The osteons are lined up along the long-axis direction and strengthen and stiffen the bone

along their length. Conversely, in the transverse plane, the less-organized matrix controls the properties of the bone.

2. Strain in a metal that is not recovered upon release of the applied load is called

    c. Plastic deformation.

    As discussed in Section 3.5, by definition the strain of a material beyond its elastic limit is plastic deformation. Unlike elastic deformation, plastic deformation is not recoverable. It is, however, very important in helping some materials resist early fracture due to repetitive loading. These concepts are discussed in Section 8.1.2.

3. With the elbow in full extension, a weight in the hand can be elevated by abduction of the whole arm. To do this, the muscle force across the shoulder must increase continually. This increasing muscle force will

    d. Increase the joint reaction force and overcome an increasing moment.

    The force of gravity remains constant as the arm is abducted, but there is an increase in the moment arm (i.e., the perpendicular distance from the line of action of the gravity force to the axis of rotation of the gleno-humeral joint). As a result, the moment produced by the gravity force increases. A close look at the mechanics of the joint (figure A.1) will show that the moment arm,

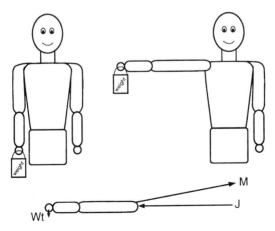

Figure A.1. A person with outstretched arm holding a weight and a free body diagram of the arm.

d, remains approximately constant as the arm is raised, so the muscle force, M, must increase in order for the opposing moment to increase. The joint reaction force, J, is nearly parallel to M, so its magnitude will be close to M. Thus both the joint reaction force and the moment will increase with abduction.

4. In mechanical characterization of a material, the change in deformation with time in response to a constant applied force is referred to as

   c. Creep

   Any response of a material that changes with time is a viscoelastic phenomenon (discussed in Section 17.1.2). By defini-

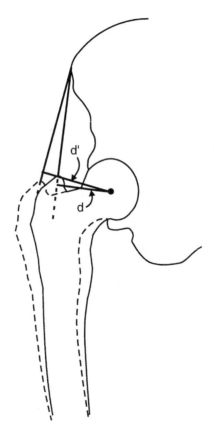

Figure A.2 Diagram of the hip showing change in moment arm with relocation of the abductor insertion on the greater tochanter.

tion, creep is the continuous deformation of a viscoelastic material over time when a constant load is applied. This is discussed in detail in Section 17.1.2.2.

5. One of the typical characteristics of a viscoelastic material is that

b. Its apparent material properties change with the rate of loading.
Any response of a material that changes with rate is also a viscoelastic phenomenon (discussed in Section 17.1). Strain-rate dependency is a viscoelastic material characteristic as discussed in Section 17.1.2.1.

6. If a prosthesis with a long neck is used in total hip arthroplasty, the distance from the abductor insertion to the center of rotation of the hip will be increased. The biomechanical consequences of this are to

c. Increase the abductor moment arm but leave the body weight moment arm unchanged.
If a long-neck prosthesis is used as shown in Figure A.2, the lateral displacement of the abductor insertion moves the line of action of the muscle away from the center of rotation of the hip joint, thus increasing the moment arm from d to d'. In addition, of course, relocation of the greater trochanter has no effect on the location of any other anatomical units.

Index

428005